Micro-irrigation System:
An Economic Analysis

Micro-irrigation System
An Economic Analysis

V.M. Rao
K. Rupkumar
J.S. Hanasashetti

ABD PUBLISHERS
Jaipur ■ New Delhi

ABD PUBLISHERS

Regd. Off. "Bony Residency", Gate No. 2
Opp. Tilak Public School, Vishweswariya Nagar,
Gopalpura Road, Jaipur - 302018, India
Ph: 0141 - 2761280, Telefax: 2761381
Email: abdpublishersjpr@gmail.com

Delhi Office: 102, 1st Floor, Satyam House,
4327/3, Ansari Road, Darya Ganj,
New Delhi - 110002, India
Ph: 011-45652440

visit us: www.oxfordbookcompany.com

Published in India, 2024

ISBN : 9788183762182

Price : ₹ 1575/-

Typeset by Shivangi Computer, Jaipur

Printed and bound in India by Thomson Press Ltd.,
New Delhi

Acknowledgements

The report is an outcome of a research project sponsored by department of agriculture, Government of Maharashtra and conducted by the Centre for Research and Publications, VAMNICOM. We are extremely thankful to Dr. Krishna Lavekar, IAS, Commissioner, Department of Agriculture, Government of Maharashtra, for entrusting the work to us. We are also thankful to Shri Bhagwati Prasad, Director of the institute for providing administrative support.

Our sincere thanks are due to Shri D.N. Gaikawad, Dy. Director Horticulture (Irrigation), and Shri J.S. Ghodke, Technical Officer, Department of Agriculture, Pune, for co-operation and arrangements made in collecting data from Latur and Osmanabad districts. Thanks are also due to Dr. S.D. Wankhede, Joint Director (Agriculture), Shri D.L. Tambhale, DSAO, Shri Bhise, SDAO, Latur, Shri D.C. Mule, SDAO, and Shri A.S. Mali, SDAO, Osmanabad for co-operation extended during field visits. We also thank all TAOs, AOs, CAOs, and other officers and supporting staff of department of agriculture in the selected districts.

An earlier version of the report was extensively reviewed by Prof. P.G. Chengappa, Vice-Chancellor, University of Agricultural Sciences, Bangalore; Prof. R.K. Sivanappan, Consultant, Coimbatore; Prof. R.S. Deshpande, Institute for Social and Economic Change, Bangalore; Prof. M. Chandrasekaran, Tamil Nadu Agricultural University, Coimbatore; Prof R.L. Shiyani, Junagadh Agricultural University, Junagadh, and Dr. A Narayanamoorthy, Gokhale Institute of Politics and Economics, Pune. We are extremely thankful to the reviewers for sparing valuable time and providing incisive comments. Efforts were made to incorporate some of the suggestions.

We would fail in our duty if we don't thank all farmers, and distributors for sparing their valuable time and sharing their feelings about micro-irrigation system.

All observations are our own, and we take responsibility for mistakes, if any.

V.M. Rao
K. Rupkumar
J.S. Hanamashetti

Preface

Irrigation remains a prime engine of agricultural growth and its importance in agricultural development has been well documented. However, water is becoming increasingly scarce. Net available potential of water for irrigation from both surface and groundwater has been declining drastically. Despite having the largest irrigated area in the world, India too has started facing severe water scarcity in different regions. Water sector will undergo dramatic changes in the years to come in order to keep with advances in technology and burgeoning population. Recognizing seriousness of the problem, GOI has taken various measures for improvement in irrigation sector. Due to rapid development of groundwater irrigation in Indian agriculture, the requirement of electricity for agriculture has also increased. In a given situation of fast declining irrigation water potential and growing demand for water, a number of demand curtailing strategies have been introduced. To increase water use efficiency especially in the use of surface irrigation water, one of the technical means introduced in Indian agriculture is Micro Irrigation System (MIS) including drip and sprinkler irrigation.

Maharashtra is one of the water scarce states and state government has been keen on promoting irrigation through

MIS by providing incentives to farmers. As a result, area covered by drip system has been substantially higher in Maharashtra compared to many other states in India.

In spite of having several advantages over the method of flood irrigation and proactive role of government owing to several reasons, progress in adoption of MIS is slow at farmers' level. In the absence of reliable field studies, it is difficult to judge the actual economic viability of MIS. At the backdrop of this, an attempt is made in the present book to assess present state and ground realties of micro irrigation at field level.

Present study is based on both secondary and primary data collected from 920 beneficiary farmers, 40 government officers, 3 manufacturers, and 8 dealers. The study covered various parameters like water saving, productivity of crops, electricity saving, fertilizer saving, economic viability of MIS, role of MIS promoters, facilitators, and administrators (Government) as well as service providers' (manufacturers and dealers) at one place.

This book will be helpful to policy makers, government officers, scholars, and general readers of agriculture. I express my sincere thanks to the M/s ABD Publishers for publishing this book in the shortest possible time for wider readership.

V.M. Rao
K. Rupkumar
J.S. Hanamashetti

Contents

1
Introduction

1.1 Overview

Water is recognized as a vital resource for life, human and societal development and environmental sustainability. However, it shows a high degree of variability in its availability, accessibility and quality. Rainfall is an inseparable and distinctive feature of India. Much of this rainfall is restricted to a few months (June-September) while the rest of the year is predominantly dry. In such a circumstance, it is only with irrigation that cultivation on an annual basis is possible. Irrigation remains a prime engine of agricultural growth and its importance in agricultural development has been well documented in India and all over world. About 70% of the world's water is used in agriculture to grow food and fibre. In developing and under development countries, it could go up to 90% while in India it is about 80% (Bhavanishankar, 2005).

Studies have confirmed that use of modern inputs, productivity of crops and intensity of cropping are significantly higher in irrigated lands compared to unirrigated lands (Vaidyanathan *et. al.*, 1994). Apart from benefiting the farmers, irrigation development also helps to increase the employment opportunities and wage rate of the agricultural landless labourers, both of which are essential to reduce poverty among them (Narayanmoorthy and Deshpande, 2003). However, water is becoming increasingly scarce.

Owing to continuous changes in cropping pattern from less water consuming crops to water intensive crops, consumption of water by agricultural sector has been increasing continuously. As a result, net available potential of water for irrigation from both surface and groundwater has been declining drastically. The rate of groundwater exploitation is going beyond socially and environmentally acceptable level in agriculturally advanced states like Punjab, Haryana, Uttar Pradesh, Tamil Nadu, etc. (Dhawan, 1995).

Despite having the largest irrigated area in the world, India too has started facing severe water scarcity in different regions. Owing to various reasons the demand for water for different purposes has been continuously increasing in India, but the potential water available for future use has been declining at a faster rate (Saleth, 1996). The agricultural sector (irrigation), which currently consumes over 80% of the available water in India, continues to be the major water-consuming sector due to the intensification of agriculture (Saleth, 1996; MOWR, 1999). Though India has the largest irrigated area in the world, the coverage of irrigation is only about 38% of the gross cropped area.

Water sector will undergo dramatic changes in the years to come in order to keep with advances in technology and burgeoning population. Much of the projected increase in demand for water will occur in developing countries, where population growth, and industrial and agricultural expansion will be greatest. It has been estimated that the water consumption by different water users will rise from 1250 Km^3/year in 1960 to about twice this amount in 2010 and to about 2800 Km^3/year in 2025. Increasing pollution of fresh water will further reduce limited fresh water (0.26% of the world's water). In addition, climate change may well cause changes in the hydrological regime, which could result in increasing stress on water resources (Ghosh and Verma, 2002).

1.2 Status of Irrigation in Maharashtra

Though Maharashtra is the most industrialized state in the country, agriculture and allied activities are still predominant in the state. About 55% of the population is dependent on agriculture for livelihood. Further, contribution of agriculture to state income is reducing from 34.4% in 1660-61 to 13.4% in 2003-04. However, for the year 1993-94 (which is base year for current national series), the corresponding share is 21.2% (GoM, 2005). Though the proportion of area under agriculture is high (57.3%) in the state as compared to national average (43.4%), agriculture is not as productive as the national level because the soil, topography and climate in Maharashtra are not much favourable to agriculture. Nearly one-third area of the state falls under rain-shadow region where rains are scanty and erratic (GoM, 2003).

Out of the total geographical area of 3.08 lakh sq. kms. of the state, area under agriculture during 2002-03 is 1.76 lakh sq. kms. In the same year, net area irrigated and gross irrigated area reported to be ha. 29.7 and ha. 36.7 lakh respectively. The percentage of gross irrigated area to gross cropped area in 2002-03 was 16.4. This percentage was 15.2 in 1990-91 and has not shown much progress during last 15 years.

The Maharashtra Water and Irrigation Commission (1999) estimated that ultimate irrigation potential of the state through both surface and groundwater resource as 1.26 lakh ha. The share of surface storages is around 85 lakh ha. A number of major, medium, and minor irrigation projects have been taken up by the state government to tap maximum possible area under irrigation. The total irrigation potential created in the state by the end of June, 2004 through these projects was 50.60 lakh ha. The share of major, medium, minor (state sectors), and minor (local sector) irrigation projects in the total irrigation potential created was 45.2%, 13.2%, 19% and 22.6% respectively. The actual utilization of irrigation potential in 2004 was 16.2 lakh ha. (32.5%) as against the potential of 49.9 lakh ha. created up to 2003 (GoM, 2005).

Recognizing seriousness of the problem, Government of Maharashtra has taken various reform measures for improvement in irrigation sector. To list a few, they are: Integrated Watershed Development Programme (1983), Irrigation Development Corporation (1996-98), Water Users Associations (2001), State Water Policy (2003), Maharashtra Water Resources Regulatory Authority Act (2003), Maharashtra Management of Irrigation System by Farmers Act (2004), etc.

1.3 Horticulture Development in Maharashtra

With the highest area under fruit crops, Maharashtra is the leading state in horticulture. State government has been implementing various programmes to promote horticulture development by establishing nurseries to supply genuine plants of various fruit crops to farmers and granting subsidy to encourage them to grow selected fruit crops. Since 1990-91, horticulture development is linked with Employment Guarantee Scheme (EGS). Up to 1990-91, area under fruit crops in the state was 2.42 lakh ha. which increased tremendously to 13.23 lakh ha. in 2004. Of the total horticultural crops, mango is cultivated on 4.25 lakh ha. followed by cashewnut 1.62 lakh ha., orange 1.30 lakh ha., pomegranate 0.85 lakh ha., sweet orange 0.84 lakh ha., banana 0.57 lakh ha., and grapes 0.39 lakh ha.

Substantial improvements in the area under horticultural crops can partly be attributed to a very high return per hectare as compared to conventional food-grain crops. Value of conventional food-grain crops is in the range of Rs. 4 thousand to Rs. 12 thousand per hectare. As against this, yield values per hectare for main fruit crops varied from Rs. 4.16 lakhs in grapes to Rs. 1.28 lakhs in mangoes (GoM, 2005). Favourable government's policies, technological innovations, better transportation and marketing options, post harvest technologies, processing units, etc., too contributed to expansion of area under these crops.

1.4 Need for Water Management

Considering the importance of irrigation in agricultural growth, prime attention has been given for the development of irrigation since independence in India. Up to 2002, about Rs. 1360.65 billion (at current prices) have been spent exclusively for the development of irrigation by the government sector, alone (Table 1.1). As a result of this, area under irrigation has increased from 26.61 mha in 1950-51 to 86.67 mha in 1996-97 (2.60% per annum). However, the share of irrigated area to GCA remained 40% as of today. But capital cost required to create one hectare of irrigation has increased substantially. As per the estimate of the Central Water Commission (CWC, 1996), India's total irrigation potential available for future use has also been declining in many states. In fact, the condition is precarious in agriculturally advanced states like Punjab, Haryana, and Tamil Nadu (Table 1.2). Further exploitation of water through Major and Medium Irrigation (MMI) and Minor Irrigation (MI) sources from these states certainly would create adverse environmental problems. Besides that, the available groundwater for use of irrigation has also been steadily declining in most of the agriculturally advanced states (Table 1.3). The principal reason for the over-exploitation of groundwater is the predominant cultivation of water intensive crops under flood method of irrigation. Therefore, cultivating crops with the present method of irrigation is no longer advisable. According to Vaidyanathan Committee Report on Pricing of Irrigation Water (GoI, 1992), the revenue collected from MMI projects is not even enough to meet the operation and maintenance cost of the irrigation system.

At the backdrop of above limitations the country has to meet various challenges. Considering the growth of population in India as well as requirements of various agricultural commodities, it is necessary to bring new area under cultivation. However, the net sown area of the country is almost constant for the last 30 years. Most of the unutilized areas are available in the form of undulating terrain and hilly areas. Recent estimates relating to future demand and supply of cereals shows that India will have cereal deficits of 36 to 64 million tonnes per year in 2020. The achievements in production of non-food-grain commodities such as oilseeds, vegetables, fruits, etc., is not also very impressive (Kumar and Mathur, 1996).

Due to rapid development of groundwater irrigation in Indian agriculture, the requirement of electricity for agriculture (irrigation pumpsets) has increased from 1982 million kwh in 1965-66 to 91277 million kwh in 1997-98. However, both water and electricity are used most inefficiently in many parts of groundwater regions because of cheaper pricing policy (either free of cost or under flat-rate tariff system) that is followed for agricultural purpose. It has certainly affected the financial position of the State Electricity Boards (SEBs). On the other hand, over-use of irrigation water causes damage to soils in the form of water logging, soil salinity, and also reduces the yield of crops (Chopra, 1996).

In a given situation of fast declining irrigation water potential and growing demand for water from different section, a number of demand curtailing strategies have been introduced since the late seventies. To increase water use efficiency especially in the use of surface irrigation water, one of the technical means introduced recently in Indian agriculture is Micro Irrigation System (MIS) including drip and sprinkler irrigation. Accordingly, irrigation efficiencies under different methods of irrigation, and advantages of drip method of irrigation over flood method have been listed in Table 1.4 and 1.5 respectively.

Table 1.1
Magnitude and Composition of Investment (Rs. crores) through Plan Periods in Irrigation and Flood Control Sectors

Plan	MMI	Minor Irrigation		Total	CAD	Flood Control	Total
		Public	Institu-tional				
First (1951-56)	376.24	65.62	Neg.				
Second (1956-61)	380.00	142.23	19.35	161.58	-	48.06	589.64
Third (1961-66)	576.00	327.73	115.37	443.10	-	82.09	1101.19
Annual (1966-69)	429.81	326.19	234.74	560.93	-	41.96	1032.70
Fourth (1969-74)	1242.30	512.28	661.06	1173.34	-	162.04	2577.68
Fifth (1974-78)	2516.18	630.83	778.76	1409.58	-	298.61	4224.38
Annual (1978-80)	2078.58	501.50	480.40	981.90	326.96	329.96	3753.40
Sixth (1980-85)	7368.83	1979.26	1437.56	3416.82	743.05	786.85	12315.55
Seventh (1985-90)	11107.29	3118.35	3060.95	6179.30	1447.50	941.58	19675.67
Annual (1990-92)	5459.15	1680.48	1349.59	3030.07	619.45	46064	9569.31
Eighth (1992-97)	21071.87	6408.36	5331.00	11739.36	2145.92	1691.68	36648.83
Ninth Plan (1997-02)*	48259.08	8615.07	2659.00	11274.07	1519.17	2629.23	63681.55
Total	100865.33	24307.90	16127.78	40435.67	6838.05	7485.91	155624.97

Note : *- anticipated: Major and Medium Irrigation; CAD – Command Area Development
Source : GOI(2002).

Table 1.2

State-wise Position of Irrigation Potential (000 ha) Created and Utilized up to IX Plan

SN	Name of State and UTs	Ultimate Irrigation Potential: MMI	MMI Potential Created Till End of IX Plan	MMI Potential Created Till End of IX Plan	Percent of Column (4) to (3)	Ultimate Irrigation Potential: MI	MI Potential Created Till End of IX Plan	MI Potential Utilized Till End of IX Plan	Percent of Column (7) to (6)
(1)	(2)	(3)	(4)	(5)	(6)	(7)	(8)	(9)	(10)
1	Andhra Pradesh	5000.00	3303.22	3051.59	66.06	6260.00	3019.46	2781.22	48.23
2	Assam	970.00	243.92	174.37	25.15	1900.00	603.62	494.11	31.77
3	Bihar	5223.50	2680.00	1714.83	51.31	5663.50	4716.44	3759.46	83.28
4	Jarkhand	1276.50	354.47	230.45	27.77	1183.50	588.87	471.09	49.76
5	Goa	62.00	21.17	15.83	34.15	54.00	19.14	20.00	35.44
6	Gujarat	3000.00	1430.37	1300.83	47.68	3103.00	1998.92	1876.14	64.42
7	Haryana	3000.00	2099.49	1849.97	69.98	1512.00	1630.95	1578.12	107.87
8	Himachal Pradesh	50.00	13.35	7.51	26.70	303.00	161.00	138.30	53.14
9	Jammu & Kashmir	250.00	179.69	168.75	71.88	1108.00	382.45	366.77	34.52
10	Karnataka	2500.00	2121.12	1844.82	84.84	3474.00	1585.40	1541.74	45.64
11	Kerala	1000.00	609.49	558.87	60.95	1679.00	640.02	603.76	38.12
12	Madhya Pradesh	4853.07	1386.90	875.63	28.58	11361.00	2256.13	2149.48	19.86
13	Chattisgarh	1146.93	922.50	760.74	80.43	571.00	487.70	322.86	85.41

(1)	(2)	(3)	(4)	(5)	(6)	(7)	(8)	(9)	(10)
14	Maharashtra	4100.00	3239.00	2147.24	79.00	4852.00	2942.60	2557.72	60.65
15	Orissa	3600.00	1826.56	1794.17	50.74	5203.00	1474.12	1337.55	28.33
16	Punjab	3000.00	2542.48	2485.99	84.75	2967.00	3427.56	3367.82	115.52
17	Rajasthan	2750.00	2482.15	2313.87	90.26	2378.00	2447.10	2361.80	102.91
18	Tamil Nadu	1500.00	1549.31	1549.29	103.29	4032.00	2123.38	2119.52	52.66
19	Uttar Pradesh	12154.00	7910.09	6334.00	65.08	17481.00	21599.40	17279.62	123.56
20	Uttaranchal	346.00	280.30	185.41	81.01	518.00	500.98	400.00	97.71
21	West Bengal	2300.00	1683.29	1527.12	73.19	4618.00	3792.52	3098.12	82.12
	Uts	98.00	6.51	3.94	6.64	46.00	43.71	35.41	95.02
	Total	58180.00	36885.38	30894.72	63.40	80267.00	56441.47	48661.41	70.32

Note : *- anticipated: Major and Medium Irrigation: CAD - Command Area Development.

Source : GOI(2002).

Table 1.3

State-wise Groundwater Potential and Development (cubic km/year)

SN	States	Total Replenishable Groundwater Reserve	Provision for Domestic, Industrial & other uses	Available Groundwater Resources for Irrigation	Net Draft	Balance Groundwater Potential Available for Exploitation	Level of Ground-water Development (%)
(1)	(2)	(3)	(4)	(5)	(6)	(7)	(8)
1	Andhra Pradesh	35.29	5.29	30.00	7.09	22.91	23.64
2	Assam	24.72	3.71	21.01	0.94	20.07	4.48
3	Bihar	33.52	5.03	28.49	5.47	23.03	19.19
4	Gujarat	20.38	3.06	17.32	7.17	10.15	41.45
5	Haryana	8.53	1.28	7.25	6.08	1.17	83.88
6	Himachal Pradesh	0.37	0.07	0.29	0.05	0.24	18.10
7	Jammu & Kashmir	4.43	0.66	3.76	0.05	3.71	1.33
8	Karnataka	6.19	2.43	13.76	4.30	9.46	31.26
9	Kerala	7.90	1.31	6.59	1.01	5.58	15.28
10	Madhya Pradesh	50.89	7.63	43.26	7.13	36.12	16.49
11	Maharashtra	37.87	12.40	25.47	7.74	17.73	30.39
12	Orissa	20.00	3.00	17.00	1.43	15.57	8.42
13	Punjab	18.66	1087	16.79	15.76	1.03	93.82

(1)	(2)	(3)	(4)	(5)	(6)	(7)	(8)
14	Rajasthan	12.71	1.99	10.71	5.42	5.29	50.63
15	Tamil Nadu	26.39	3.96	22.43	13.56	8.87	60.44
16	Uttar Pradesh	83.82	12.57	71.25	26.84	44.41	37.67
17	West Bengal	23.09	3.46	19.63	4.75	14.88	24.18
	All States	431.48	70.74	360.74	115.01	245.73	31.88
	All UTs	0.41	0.19	0.21	0.17	0.06	76.19
	All India	431.89	70.93	360.96	115.17	245.79	31.92

Note : Total may not tally due to rounding off figures.
Source: CWC (1998).

Table 1.4
Irrigation Efficiencies (%) under Different Methods of Irrigation

Irrigation Efficiencies	Methods of Irrigation		
	Surface	Sprinkler	Drip
Conveyance efficiency	40-50 (canal) 60-70 (well)	100	100
Application efficiency	60-70	70-80	90
Surface water moisture evaporation	30-40	30-40	20-25
Overall efficiency	30-35	50-60	80-90

Source : Sivanappan (1998).

Table 1.5
Comparative Advantages of Drip irrigation over Flood Irrigation

SN	Variables	Drip Method	Flood Method
1	Water saving	40-100 percent	Less owing to evaporation
2	Irrigation efficiency	80-90 percent	30-50 percent
3	Input cost	Less especially in labour, fertilizers, pesticides and tilling	Comparatively higher
4	Weed problem	Reduced significantly	Very High
5	Suitable water	Even saline water can be used	Only normal water can be used
6	Diseases and pest problems	Relatively less	High/moderate
7	Water logging	Nil	About 8.5 mha is under water logging in India
8	Water control	Easily manageable	Difficult to manage
9	Evaporation and transportation losses	Very low	Very high
10	Labor requirement	Relatively low	High
11	Efficiency of fertilizer use	Very high and constant supply	Heavy losses owing to leaching and evaporation
12	B-C ratio	Excluding water saving: 1.3-13.3 including water saving: 2.8-30.0	In the range of 1.8-3.9

13	Capital cost/ha	Rs. 15000-40000 varies with space and crops	Rs. 70000 for MMI projects during 7th plan
14	Product quality	Relatively better	Normal
15	Increase in yield	About 20-100 percent higher vis-à-vis flood method	Yield is less compared to drip irrigation

Source: Narayanamoorthy (2005).

Since drip irrigation is a new technology and capital intensive, government operates a scheme with subsidy. Though a central scheme was started in 1982-83 by Ministry of Water Resources, it was extended to Maharashtra in 1991-92. Government of Maharashtra has also been providing subsidy under state scheme from 1986-87. Details of progress made in MIS by the state have been given in Chapter 2.

1.5 Need for the Study

Maharashtra is one of the water scarce states in India. Area under irrigation in the state is hovering between 15 to 16% of gross cropped area (GCA) from last 15 years, which is quite low. Moreover, horticultural crops like grapes, pomegranate, banana, etc., are also being extensively cultivated in the state under drip irrigation. State government is also keen on promoting irrigation through drip system by providing subsidies for farmers. Importantly, area covered by drip system is substantially higher in Maharashtra compared to many other states in India. On the other hand, existing groundwater exploitation of Maharashtra is only 24% of the recharge (Dhawan, 1995), and well irrigation is most suitable source of efficient utilization of drip irrigation, remaining potential of groundwater can be shifted under MIS. Besides that there is need for shifting of sugarcane area under drip irrigation in order to save and more efficient use of scarce water resource. Above points clearly indicate need for study of the problems and prospects of MIS.

1.6 Rationale of the Study

Though drip irrigated area has been consistently increasing in Maharashtra, trends in development of drip area are not same across different districts. The rate of increase is well above state average (254) in divisions like Nashik (667), Aurangabad (802), and Latur (327) between 1986-87 to 1994-95, while it is less in Konkan and Nagpur divisions (Narayanmoorthy, 1996).

Development of MIS is determined by factors like availability and quality of surface water sources, groundwater development, pattern of crop, economic conditions of the farmers, rainfall, area under commercial and wide spaced crops, type of farmers, structure of farming (commercial or subsistence), availability of extension services, and policy of government. It is obvious that these determining factors widely vary across districts and regions. Hence, it is important to understand district-wise development of drip and sprinkler irrigation. Besides this, owing to technical aspects involved in efficient functioning of the system on one hand and ignorance of farmers on the other hand leads to many operational problems and ultimately result in the partial and/ or non-use of installed MI sets. Such cases are noticed by GoM in various districts of Maharashtra. Keeping in view these important considerations and future perspective, the study was undertaken purposively in Latur and Osmanabad districts of Maharashtra to explore the ground realities at micro-level.

1.7 District Profiles of Latur and Osmanabad Districts

1.7.1 Agro-climatic

Latur and Osmanabad districts are situated to the east of Marathwada region of the state. Geographically, Latur district covered 2.32% and Osmanabad 2.43% area of the state. Agro-climatic zone-wise these two districts fall under 'assured rainfall zone' and partly in 'scarcity zone' (Osmanabad district). Soils of these districts range from deep black soils to medium black soils. Climate is tropical rainy, maximum and minimum temperature varies between 42^{0}C to 8^{0}C while average annual rainfall received by them ranges between 500 to 600 mm. The adversities imposed by the inadequate, seasonal, and erratic rainfall impose several constraints on speedy development of agriculture in the districts.

1.7.2 *Land Use Details*

Of the respective geographical area of Latur and Osmanabad districts, net sown area accounted about 75% and 68% respectively. Percentage of net irrigated area to the respective GCA varied from 6% in Latur to 13% in Osmanabad. This depicts the dismal picture of the districts on irrigation front. On the other hand, culturable waste land is worked out as much as 14% and 20% of the respective GCA of Latur and Osmanabad districts which could be brought under cultivation with suitable technology adoption.

1.7.3 *Cropping Pattern*

Assured rainfall and deep black soils are the important resources of the districts. Crops are being grown in both kharif and rabi seasons. Cropping pattern of both the districts dominated by food-grains and accounted about 65% and 72% of the respective GCA in Latur and Osmanabad district respectively. Major crops grown in the districts are jowar, bajara, and wheat as cereals, tur, gram, and urid as pulses, and sunflower, safflower, and groundnut as oilseeds. Among cash crops, sugarcane and cotton are important. Mango, grapes, pomegranate, and guava are the important fruit crops being grown in the districts. However, total area under fruits and vegetables hovered around 1% to 2% in the districts. Cropping pattern of the districts experienced gradual shift in favour of sunflower, sugarcane, fruits, and vegetables.

1.8 Objectives of the Study

In spite of having several advantages over the method of flood irrigation and proactive role of GoM, adoption of MIS is slow at farmers' level. In the absence of reliable field studies, it is difficult to judge the actual economic viability of MIS. Thus, an attempt is made in the present study to assess state and ground realities of micro-irrigation at farm level in order to draw exemplary lessons, as also to identify associated problems/constraints in implementation and ways and means of resolving them. Specific objectives of the study are:

1. To examine present status and prospects of micro-irrigation system (drip/sprinkler) in the context of changing cropping pattern in Latur and Osmanabad districts,
2. to analyse performance of micro-irrigation system at field level in regard to costs, returns, and economic viability of selected crops,
3. to evaluate impact of micro-irrigation on input-use, production, and productivity of selected crops under micro-irrigation,
4. to study the role and scope of government agencies, manufacturers, and dealers in promoting micro-irrigation in the districts, and
5. to study various operational/financial/administrative problems faced by respondents in adopting technology, and suggest measures for their minimization.

1.9 Methodology Adopted

The study utilizes both secondary and primary data. Secondary data pertaining to adoption of number of drip sets and sprinkler sets, crop-wise area covered under these systems of irrigation, and subsidy granted were collected from various published and unpublished sources, and various offices for the period of 1986-87 to 2004-05 (Tables 1.6 to 1.15).

It is clear from Table 1.15 that there are as many as 6430 drip farmers and 2770 sprinkler farmers in Latur and Osmanabad districts during 2001-05. In the first stage, taluka-wise as also village-wise list of farmers adopting both drip and sprinklers were prepared. Secondly, from each selected village all households having land were listed on the basis of farm size of holdings in ascending order. Thirdly, households were divided into marginal (less than ha.1), small (ha.1-2),

Table 1.6 (a)

Assistance Provided for Drip and Sprinklers in Latur and Osmanabad Districts, 2001-05

S.N.	Year	Latur			
		Drip		Sprinkler	
		Physical (ha)	Assistance (lakhs)	Physical (ha)	Assistance (lakhs)
1	2000-01	216.38	40.12	513	46.17
2	2001-02	766.79	110.92	977	124.03
3	2002-03	38.45	21.24	363	37.90
4	2003-04	309.95	22.75	346	20.76
5	2004-05	34.06	3.06	43	2.58
	Total	1365.63	198.09	2242	231.44

Table 1.6 (b)

Assistance Provided for Drip and Sprinklers in Latur and Osmanabad Districts, 2001-05

S.N.	Year	Osmanabad			
		Drip		Sprinkler	
		Physical (ha)	Assistance (lakhs)	Physical (ha)	Assistance (lakhs)
1	2000-01	216.38	40.12	513	46.17
1	2000-01	726.34	178.14	202	23.29
2	2001-02	416.26	76.51	2	0.24
3	2002-03	3625.61	679.19	163	19.26
4	2003-04	226.01	21.15	156	8.76
5	2004-05	75.80	5.38	5	0.21
	Total	5070.02	960.37	528	51.76

Source: JDA Office, Latur.

Table 1.7
Taluka-wise Distribution of Area Covered (ha.) under Drip in Latur District, 2001-05

S.N.	Taluka	2000-01	2001-02	2002-03	2003-04	2004-05	Total
1	Latur	65.2	110.72	30.35	101.91	2.8	310.98
2	Renapur	37.89	65.18	0.36	89.48	2.66	195.57
3	Ausa	48.25	20.7	6.03	85.48	11.49	171.95
4	Nilanga	13.5	12.27	0.4	24.52	3.49	54.18
5	Udgir	17.31	231.87	0.55	0	3.19	252.92
6	Jalkot	1.41	15.33	0	0	0.47	17.21
7	Deonee	3.09	47.71	0	0	0.33	51.13
8	Ahmadpur	4.72	36.04	0.4	0	2.05	43.21
9	Chakur	20.32	226.97	0.36	8.56	6.1	262.31
10	Shirur	4.69	0	0	0	1.48	0
	Total	216.38	766.79	38.45	309.95	34.06	1365.63

Source: JDA Office, Latur.

Table 1.8
Taluka-wise Distribution of Sample under Drip in Latur District, 2001-05

S.N.	Taluka	2000-01	2001-02	2002-03	2003-04	2004-05	Total
1	Latur	7	11	3	10	0	31
2	Renapur	4	7	0	9	0	20
3	Ausa	5	2	1	8	1	17
4	Nilanga	1	1	0	2	1	5
5	Udgir	2	23	0	0	0	25
6	Jalkot	0	2	0	0	0	2
7	Devanee	0	5	0	0	0	5
8	Ahmadpur	0	4	0	0	0	4
9	Chakur	2	22	0	1	1	26
10	Shirur	1	0	0	0	0	1
	Total	22	77	4	30	3	136

Source: JDA Office, Latur.

Table 1.9

Taluka-wise Distribution of Area Covered (ha.) under Sprinklers in Latur District, 2001-05

S.N.	Taluka	2000-01	2001-02	2002-03	2003-04	2004-05	Total
1	Latur	121.02	335.70	73.07	62.42	11.81	604.02
2	Renapur	120.25	555.23	74.31	141.69	4.44	895.92
3	Ausa	84.95	21.49	0	100.16	5.90	212.5
4	Nilanga	67.46	64.58	9.73	41.73	7.36	190.86
5	Udgir	19.54	0	36.55	0	2.12	58.21
6	Jalkot	4.62	0	0	0	0.77	5.39
7	Devanee	3.90	0	0	0	0.65	4.55
8	Ahmadpur	24.62	0	47.52	0	2.62	74.76
9	Chakur	47.14	0	119.39	0	4.13	170.66
10	Shirur	19.50	0	2.43	0	3.20	25.13
	Total	513	977	363	346	43	2242

Source: JDA Office, Latur.

Table 1.10

Taluka-wise Distribution of Sample under Sprinklers in Latur District, 2001-05

S.N.	Taluka	2000-01	2001-02	2002-03	2003-04	2004-05	Total
1	Latur	12	34	7	6	2	61
2	Renapur	12	56	7	15	0	90
3	Ausa	8	2	0	10	1	21
4	Nilanga	7	6	1	4	1	19
5	Udgir	2	0	4	0	0	6
6	Jalkot	1	0	0	0	0	1
7	Devanee	0	0	0	0	0	0
8	Ahmadpur	2	0	5	0	0	7
9	Chakur	5	0	12	0	0	17
10	Shirur	2	0	0	0	0	2
	Total	51	98	36	39	4	224

Source: JDA Office, Latur.

Table 1.11
Taluka-wise Distribution of Area Covered (ha.) under Drip in Osmanabad District, 2001-05

S.N.	Taluka	2000-01	2001-02	2002-03	2003-04	2004-05	Total
1	Tuljapur	70.67	68.97	0	70.06	18.93	228.63
2	Osmanabad	291.92	268.20	1223.64	53.93	9.41	1847.10
3	Umarga	15.76	0	0	14.06	9.47	39.29
4	Lohara	0	0	0	0	8.66	8.66
5	Bhoom	31.45	10.24	68.89	33.02	12.10	155.70
6	Paranda	32.54	9.95	147.20	23.75	5.48	218.92
7	Kalamb	284	58.90	2185.88	24.36	8.78	2561.92
8	Washi	0	0	0	6.83	2.97	9.80
	Total	726.34	416.26	3625.61	226.01	75.8	5070.02

Source: JDA Office, Latur.

Table 1.12
Taluka-wise Distribution of Sample under Drip in Osmanabad District, 2001-05

S.N.	Taluka	2000-01	2001-02	2002-03	2003-04	2004-05	Total
1	Tuljapur	07	07	00	07	02	23
2	Osmanabad	29	27	122	06	01	185
3	Umarga	01	00	00	01	01	03
4	Lohara	00	00	00	00	01	01
5	Bhoom	03	01	07	04	01	16
6	Paranda	04	01	15	02	00	22
7	Kalamb	28	06	219	02	01	256
8	Washi	00	00	00	01	00	01
	Total	72	42	363	23	07	507

Source: JDA Office, Latur

Table 1.13
Taluka-wise Distribution of Area Covered (ha.) under Sprinklers in Osmanabad District, 2001-05

S.N.	Taluka	2000-01	2001-02	2002-03	2003-04	2004-05	Total
1	Tuljapur	39.51	0.60	00	45.00	0.34	85.45
2	Osmanabad	65.93	0.08	135.29	31.50	2.10	234.90
3	Umarga	36.56	0.77	00	30.78	0.29	68.40
4	Lohara	00	.00	00	5.02	00	5.02
5	Bhoom	14.62	00	13.21	13.35	0.48	41.66
6	Paranda	7.76	00	00	8.62	0.33	16.71
7	Kalamb	37.62	0.55	9.81	21.73	1.46	71.17
8	Washi	00	00	4.69	00	00	4.69
	Total	202	02	163	156	05	528

Source: JDA Office, Latur.

Table 1.14
Taluka-wise Distribution of Sample under Sprinklers in Osmanabad District, 2001-05

S.N.	Taluka	2000-01	2001-02	2002-03	2003-04	2004-05	Total
1	Tuljapur	04	00	00	05	00	09
2	Osmanabad	06	00	14	03	00	23
3	Umarga	04	00	00	03	00	07
4	Lohara	00	00	00	01	00	01
5	Bhoom	02	00	01	01	00	04
6	Paranda	01	00	0	01	00	02
7	Kalamb	04	00	01	02	00	07
8	Washi	00	00	00	00	00	00
	Total	21	00	16	16	00	53

Source: JDA Office, Latur.

Table 1.15
Sample Size

S.N.	Particular	Latur	Osmanabad	Total
1	Area covered (in Ha.) under drip during 2000-05	1360	5070	6430
2	10% sample	136	507	643
3	Total sample size for drip	643		
4	Area covered (1 set = 1 Ha) under sprinkler during 2000-05	2242	528	2770
5	10% sample	224	53	277
6	Total sample size for sprinkler	277		
	Final Sample Size	920		

Source: Dy. Director (Irrigation), Commissionerate of Agriculture, GoM, Pune.

medium (ha. 2-4), and large (more than ha. 4). Finally, n^{th} household from this list was selected for detailed investigation. Size of n for each village was calculated roughly by dividing total number of households in a particular village by number of households to be surveyed from that village. A moderate sample of 10% from total area covered under drip and sprinkler during 2001-05 were selected. Thus, a total sample of 920 farmers covering 643 from drip and 277 from sprinkler were selected.

Primary data on various parameters (age, education, social group, land holding, cropping pattern, cost of cultivation, annual income, source of information, problems faced, expectations, etc.) were collected with the help of specially structured survey schedules through personal interview method. Field visits were undertaken during November 2006 to January 2007 in 18 blocks of both the districts (10 blocks of Latur district and 8 blocks of Osmanabad district).

On the basis of highest concentration of area, sugarcane and grapes under drip, and sugarcane and gram under sprinkler were identified as crops to be studied to evaluate the impact of respective methods of irrigation at farm level. Sample farmers were asked to provide data on relative expenses incurred on selected crops under drip/sprinkler technology vis-à-vis traditional method of irrigation, before and after approach was followed.

As a promoter, facilitator, and administrator, state government is playing crucial role in MIS implementation in the state. An attempt is also made to study the role and scope of government agencies as well as various problems encountered by them in effective implementation of MIS. Accordingly, 40 officers across rank and file (Sub-Divisional Agriculture Officer to Circle Agriculture Officer) from both the districts were personally interviewed. Required data was collected through specially designed schedules.

Apart from government agencies, service-providers, namely, MI manufacturers and dealers are playing important role in supply of BIS standard quality materials and support services in addition to MIS promotion, popularization, and extension activities. Experiences learned by them at field level bears significant importance in greater technical and satisfactory services to the MIS adopters. Besides this, further horizontal penetration of MIS on geographical basis greatly depends on efforts and services put by MIS service providers. Keeping in view of this, 3 major manufacturers, and 8 MIS dealers (4 each from Latur and Osmanabad district) representing various companies were visited personally to collect required data. Separate schedules were designed for this purpose.

Thus, present study is an attempt to cover present status and problems of all stakeholders (beneficiary-farmers, government officers, manufacturers, and dealers) of micro-irrigation system at one place.

1.10 Organization of the Study

The study has been divided into 8 chapters. Chapter 1 deals with an overview of water scenario, need for water management, need for the study, rationale of the study, objectives, profile of selected districts, methodology adopted, and criteria for selection of sample and crops. While present status of MIS at national vis-à-vis state and study districts level forms the part of Chapter 2, analytical details of performance of MIS at farmers level with respect to various socio-economical and techno-feasibility parameters followed by critical discussions are given in Chapter 3. Further, Chapter 4 presents the impact of micro-irrigation on input-use performance at micro-level. Importance of government agencies, manufacturers, and MIS dealers in the context of assigned roles in implementation of MIS have been analyzed and the arrived results are provided in Chapters 5, 6, and 7 respectively. Operational/financial/administrative problems faced by respondents are discussed in Chapter 8. The last and final Chapter 9 summarizes the study findings and provide policy implications to the concerned for effective implementation of MIS in the state.

2

Status of MIS in Latur and Osmanabad Districts

This chapter analyzes the increase in area under drip/sprinkler irrigation in India as well as in Maharashtra state. Further, an attempt is also made to reveal district-wise area under drip/sprinkler irrigation in the state.

2.1 Drip Irrigation in Maharashtra

In the early seventies, agricultural universities and other research institutions introduced drip irrigation in India. During initial years the development was very slow, but significant development has been achieved in the recent years. Though India has enormous potential and prospects, the development of drip irrigation is not impressive in most of the states. Table 2.1 presents state-wise area under drip method of irrigation and its growth rate for two time points: 1991-92 and 1997-98. The table denotes that drip irrigated area has increased substantially between the early nineties and late nineties in all the states in India. Maharashtra state alone accounted for nearly 50% of India's total drip irrigated area followed by Karnataka (16.58%), Tamil Nadu (13.86%), and Andhra Pradesh (10.70%).

Table 2.1
State-wise Area (ha.) under Drip Irrigation

S.N.	State	Area		%		ACGR
		1991-92	1997-98	1991-92	1997-98	(Area)
1	Maharashtra	32924	122995[a]	44.64	50	24.56
2	Karnataka	11412	40800[b]	16.17	16.58	23.66
3	Tamil Nadu	5357	34100	7.59	13.86	36.14
4	Abdhra Pradesh	11585	26300	16.41	10.7	14.64
5	Gujarat	3560	7000	5.05	2.85	11.93
6	Kerala	3035	4865	4.3	1.98	8.18
7	Orissa	44	2696	0.06	1.1	98.55
8	Haryana	120	1900	0.17	0.77	58.46
9	Rajasthan	304	1600	0.43	0.65	31.89
10	Uttar Pradesh	111	1500	0.16	0.61	54.33
11	Punjab	20	1100	0.03	0.45	85.01
12	Other states	2117	1150	3	0.47	-9.67
	Total	70589	246006	100	100	23.13

Source : AFC, 1998.

Note: a = includes State subsidy scheme area of 58498 ha. and b = includes area under Central and State schemes for development of oil palm and sugarcane.
ACGR = Annual compound growth rate per cent per annum between 1991-92 and 1997-98

Over the last ten years, significant growth has been achieved in area under drip method of irrigation in many states. Despite significant growth in area under drip method of irrigation, drip irrigated area constitutes a very meagre percentage in relation to gross irrigated area in all the states of India. Lack of awareness and less popularity among the farmers about the advantage of drip irrigation are the main reasons for the less development of drip irrigation in India.

2.2 District-wise Development of Drip Irrigation

The trends in development of area under drip are not same across different districts of the state even though the drip irrigated area has been consistently increasing in Maharashtra. Factors such as availability of water (surface and ground), cropping pattern, farmers' economic condition, rainfall, area under commercial crops, structure of farming, availability of extension services and government's policy determine the development of drip irrigation. It is apparent that these decisive factors widely differ across districts and regions. An attempt has been made to analyze district-wise and region-wise development of drip irrigated area across Maharashtra during 1987 to 2005.

Table 2.2 depicts district-wise area under drip irrigation and its district-wise proportion to total area in the state. It is clear from table that area under drip irrigation in Maharashtra has consistently increased from 237 ha. in 1987 to 36958 ha. in 2005, implying a rise of 156 times during the 18 years period. But, development of drip is not uniform across the districts.

The rate of increase in area covered under drip is high in divisions like Nashik, Pune, and Aurangabad, on the other hand, it is less in divisions like Nagpur and Amravati. For example, the rate of increase is about 511 times in Nashik, 130 times in Pune and 315 in Aurangabad between 1987 to 2005, while the same is only 155 times in the state as a whole during above mentioned period. Mainly two phenomena are responsible for the rapid increase of drip irrigated area (Nashik, Pune and Aurangabad). Firstly, crops which are suitable for drip irrigation are extensively cultivated and secondly, due to depletion of groundwater and scarcity of water, farmers have installed drip system as water saving technology. But in case of Nagpur and Amarawati they grow crops, which are not suitable for drip irrigation; therefore growth of drip irrigation is not impressive (Narayanmoorthy, 1996).

2.3 District-wise Subsidy Disbursement

For promotion of drip irrigation state scheme is in operation since 1986-87. Data related to area under drip irrigation and amount of subsidy disbursed during 1986-95 and 2000-05 is explained in Table 2.3. Total area of drip irrigation under state and central schemes together was 60130 ha. and 127453 ha. during 1986-95 and 2000-05 respectively. In the same fashion, the amount of subsidy disbursed was Rs. 8372 lakhs and Rs. 13622 lakhs respectively. It is also worth to notify that, the percentage change in area and subsidy between 1986-95 and 2000-05 were 111.96% and 62.71% respectively. Across divisions, Latur division has registered highest percentage change (114.56%) in subsidy disbursement during above-mentioned period. This is followed by Pune (96.69%), Nashik (79.44%). However, Konkan division registered negative growth in disbursement of subsidy during 1986-95 to 2000-05.

2.4 Sprinkler Irrigation in Maharashtra

Similar to drip method of irrigation, sprinkler irrigation is also an advanced water saving technology predominantly used in Western countries. Sprinkler irrigation is a relatively old technology for Indian farmers when compared to the drip irrigation method. States like Haryana, Rajasthan, and Madhya Pradesh initially started using the sprinkler method of irrigation. Unlike drip method, narrow spaced crops such as wheat, sugarcane, oilseeds, pulse millets, cotton, vegetables, coffee, tea, etc., are highly suitable for the application of the sprinkler irrigation method.

Though Maharashtra accounts for over 50% of India's total drip irrigated area as of today, its share in sprinkler irrigation comes to only about 5% (INCID, 1998). District-wise area covered and numbers of sprinkler sets distributed are given in Table 2.4. As per the data available from GoM, the area under sprinkler and number of sprinkler sets decreased from 14972.97 ha. and 16043 in 2000-01 to 7789.56 ha. and 8012 respectively in 2003-04. As the numbers of sprinkler sets distributed were decreased, the area under sprinkler irrigation also declined. Across divisions in Maharashtra, Nasik, Pune, Kolhapur and Aurangabad registered increase

Table 2.2
District-wise Area (ha.) under Drip Irrigation

S.N.	District	1987	1991	1995	2001	2002	2003	2004	2005
1	Thane	1	102	182	-	94	-	17	160
		(0.42)	(1.60)	(1.37)		(0.63)		(0.08)	(0.43)
2	Raigad	-	15	45	-	27	31	-	73
			(0.24)	(0.34)		(0.18)	(0.07)		(0.20)
3	Ratnagiri	3	12	62	102	84	35	35	469
		(1.27)	(0.19)	(0.47)	(0.86)	(0.57)	(0.08)	(0.18)	(1.27)
4	Sindhudurg	1	35	58	-	141	132	88	34
		(0.42)	(0.55)	(0.44)		(0.95)	(0.3)	(0.45)	(0.1)
Konkan		5	164	347	102	346	198	140	736
		(2.11)	(2.58)	(2.62)	(0.86)	(2.33)	(0.45)	(0.71)	(2.00)
5	Nashik	16	1529	2538	1877	1238	5563	4339	8611
		(6.75)	(24.01)	(19.17)	(15.8)	(8.33)	(12.62)	(22.05)	(23.3)
6	Dhule	-	21	184	519	434	1789	416	411
			(0.33)	(1.39)	(4.37)	(2.92)	(4.06)	(2.12)	(1.11)
7	Nandurbar	-	-	-	280	110	587	152	126
					(2.36)	(0.74)	(1.33)	(0.77)	(0.34)
8	Jalgaon	10	356	1818	1787	1281	10546	2922	4145
		(4.22)	(5.59)	(13.73)	(15.04)	(8.62)	(23.92)	(14.85)	(11.22)
Nashik		26	1906	4540	4463	3063	18485	7829	13293
		(10.97)	(29.93)	(34.29)	(37.57)	(20.61)	(41.93)	(39.79)	(35.97)
9	Ahmednagar	20	627	800	649	1394	1824	1452	2150
		(8.44)	(9.85)	(6.04)	(5.47)	(9.38)	(4.14)	(7.38)	(5.82)

10	Pune	15 (6.33)	256 (4.02)	1237 (9.35)	462 (3.89)	674 (4.54)	1766 (4.01)	926 (4.71)	1755 (4.75)
11	Solapur	55 (23.2)	287 (4.50)	1225 (9.25)	1382 (11.63)	1651 (11.11)	6186 (14.03)	1929 (9.8)	7780 (21.05)
Pune		90 (37.97)	1170 (18.37)	3262 (24.64)	2493 (20.99)	3719 (25.03)	9776 (22.18)	4307 (21.89)	11685 (31.62)
12	Satara	4 (1.69)	95 (1.49)	230 (1.74)	300 (2.53)	163 (1.1)	373 (0.85)	105 (0.53)	713 (1.93)
13	Sangli	36 (15.19)	238 (3.74)	608 (4.59)	1345 (11.32)	1024 (6.89)	2135 (4.84)	1857 (9.44)	2716 (7.34)
14	Kolhapur	7 (2.95)	151 (2.37)	120 (0.91)	107 (0.9)	167 (1.12)	106 (0.24)	116 (0.59)	368 (1.00)
Kolhapur		47 (19.83)	484 (7.60)	958 (7.24)	1752 (14.75)	1354 (9.11)	2614 (5.93)	2078 (10.56)	3797 (10.27)
15	Aurangabad	-	532 (8.36)	560 (4.23)	906 (7.63)	1340 (9.02)	1878 (4.26)	1029 (5.23)	1354 (3.66)
16	Jalna	4 (1.69)	162 (2.54)	345 (2.6)	282 (2.37)	535 (3.6)	618 (1.4)	968 (4.92)	702 (1.90)
17	Beed	3 (1.27)	62 (0.97)	189 (1.43)	190 (1.6)	154 (1.04)	347 (0.79)	297 (1.51)	148 (0.40)
Aurangabad		7 (2.96)	756 (11.87)	1094 (8.26)	1378 (11.6)	2029 (13.66)	2843 (6.45)	2294 (11.66)	2204 (5.96)
18	Latur	3 (1.27)	240 (3.77)	230 (1.74)	216 (1.82)	767 (5.16)	38 (0.08)	310 (1.58)	464 (1.25)
19	Osmanabad	12 (5.06)	132 (2.07)	157 (1.18)	726 (6.11)	416 (2.80)	3626 (8.23)	226 (1.15)	946 (2.56)

S.N.	District	1987	1991	1995	2001	2002	2003	2004	2005
20	Nanded	2 (0.84)	304 (4.77)	369 (2.79)	161 (1.35)	134 (0.9)	705 (1.6)	600 (3.05)	931 (2.52)
21	Hingoli	-	-	-	146 (1.23)	184 (1.24)	282 (0.64)	220 (1.12)	258 (0.78)
22	Parbhani	4 (1.69)	210 (3.3)	539 (4.07)	204 (1.72)	478 (3.22)	761 (1.73)	304 (1.54)	361 (0.98)
Latur		21 (8.86)	886 (13.91)	1295 (9.78)	1453 (12.23)	1979 (13.32)	5412 (12.28)	1660 (8.44)	2960 (8.01)
23	Buldhana	2 (0.84)	171 (2.69)	140 (1.06)	15 (0.13)	264 (1.78)	1103 (2.5)	299 (1.52)	412 (1.11)
24	Akola	3 (1.27)	149 (2.34)	208 (1.57)	-	391 (2.63)	313 (0.71)	117 (0.59)	93 (0.25)
25	Washim	-	-	-	-	103 (0.69)	261 (0.59)	91 (0.46)	104 (0.28)
26	Amravati	6 (2.53)	350 (5.50)	315 (2.38)	5 (0.04)	647 (4.35)	2092 (4.75)	458 (2.33)	1351 (3.66)
27	Yavatmal	10 (4.22)	155 (2.43)	197 (1.49)	-	361 (2.43)	322 (0.73)	39 (0.2)	99 (0.27)
Amravati		21 (8.86)	825 (12.96)	860 (6.5)	20 (0.17)	1766 (11.88)	4091 (9.28)	1004 (5.1)	2059 (5.57)
28	Wardha	9 (3.8)	90 (1.41)	279 (2.11)	217 (1.83)	155 (1.04)	109 (0.25)	74 (0.38)	37 (0.10)
29	Nagpur	9 (3.80)	51 (0.80)	106 (0.80)	-	414 (2.79)	511 (1.16)	257 (1.31)	167 (0.46)

30	Bhandara	-	22 (0.35)	15 (0.11)	-	14 (0.10)	14 (0.03)	6 (0.03)	2 (NG)
31	Gondia	-	-	-	-	20 (0.13	27 (0.06	12 (0.06	3 (NG)
32	Chandrapur	2 (0.84)	8 (0.13)	6 (0.05)	-	-	2 (NG)	13 (0.06)	14 (0.04)
33	Gadchiroli	-	6 (0.09)	1 (NG)	-	-	-	2 (0.01)	1 (NG)
Nagpur		20 (8.44)	177 (2.78)	407 (3.07)	217 (1.83)	603 (4.06)	663 (1.50)	364 (1.85)	224 (0.60)
Demonstration		w-	-	476 (3.60)	-	-	-	-	-
Maharashtra		237 (100.00)	6368 (100.00)	13239 (100.00)	11878 (100.00)	14859 (100.00)	44082 (100.00)	19676 (100.00)	36958 (100.00)

Source : Narayanamoorthy, 1996 and Commissionerate of Agriculture, Pune.

Table 2.3
District-wise Area (ha.) and Subsidy (Rs. lakh) under Drip Irrigation

S.N.	District	1986-1995		2000-2005		% change	
		Area	Subsidy	Area	Subsidy	Area	Subsidy
1	Thane	1174 (1.95)	88 (1.05)	271 (0.21)	24 (0.18)	-76.29	-72.73
2	Raigad	159 (0.26)	14 (0.17)	131 (0.1)	9 (0.07)	-17.61	-35.71
3	Ratnagiri	198 (0.33)	23 (0.27)	725 (0.57)	29 (0.21)	266.16	26.09
4	Sindhudurg	334 (0.56)	31 (0.37)	395 (0.31)	22 (0.16)	18.26	-29.03
Konkan		1865 (3.1)	156 (1.86)	1522 (1.19)	84 (0.62)	-18.39	-46.15
5	Nashik	10938 (18.19)	1590 (18.99)	21628 (16.97)	1973 (14.48)	97.73	24.09
6	Dhule	915 (1.52)	128 (1.53)	3569 (2.80)	490 (3.60)	290.05	282.81
7	Nandurbar	-	-	1255 (0.98)	196 (1.44)		
8	Jalgaon	5375 (8.94)	953 (11.38)	20681 (16.23)	2134 (15.66)	284.76	123.92
Nashik		17228 (28.65)	2671 (31.90)	47133 (36.98)	4793 (35.18)	173.58	79.44

9	Ahmednagar	5210 (8.67)	713 (8.52)	7469 (5.86)	928 (6.82)	43.36	30.15
10	Pune	3676 (6.11)	464 (5.54)	5583 (4.38)	679 (4.98)	51.87	46.34
11	Solapur	4664 (7.76)	636 (7.60)	18928 (14.85)	1959 (14.38)	305.83	208.02
Pune		13550 (22.54)	1813 (21.66)	31980 (25.09)	3566 (26.18)	136.01	96.69
12	Satara	1421 (2.36)	216 (2.58)	1654 (1.30)	187 (1.37)	16.4	-13.42
13	Sangli	3288 (5.47)	559 (6.68)	9077 (7.12)	981 (7.20)	176.06	75.49
14	Kolhapur	1223 (2.04)	174 (2.07)	864 (0.68)	85 (0.63)	-29.35	-51.15
Kolhapur		5932 (9.87)	949 (11.33)	11595 (9.10)	1253 (9.20)	95.46	32.03
15	Aurangabad	3377 (5.62)	400 (4.78)	6507 (5.10)	522 (3.83)	92.68	30.5
16	Jalna	1535 (2.55)	186 (2.22)	3105 (2.44)	297 (2.18)	102.28	59.68
17	Beed	943 (1.57)	123 (1.47)	1136 (0.89)	107 (0.79	20.46	-13.01
Aurangabad		5855 (9.74)	709 (8.47)	10748 (8.43)	926 (6.80)	83.57	30.61
18	Latur	2050 (3.41)	248 (2.96)	1795 (1.41)	236 (1.73)	-12.44	-4.84

S.N.	District	1986-1995		2000-2005		% change	
		Area	Subsidy	Area	Subsidy	Area	Subsidy
19	Osmanabad	937	132	5940	1005	533.94	661.36
		(1.56)	(1.58)	(4.66)	(7.38)		
20	Nanded	1800	226	2531	273	40.61	20.79
		(2.99)	(2.70)	(1.99)	(2.00)		
21	Hingoli	-	-	1090	117		
				(0.86)	(0.86)		
22	Parbhani	1926	266	2108	240	9.45	-9.77
		(3.20)	(3.18)	(1.65)	(1.76)		
Latur			6713	872	13464	1871	100.56
		114.56					
		(11.16)	(10.42)	(10.57)	(13.73)		
23	Buldhana	1419	140	2093	316	47.5	125.71
		(2.36)	(1.67)	(1.64)	(2.32)		
24	Akola	1269	142	914	81	-27.97	-42.96
		(2.11)	(1.70)	(0.72)	(0.60)		
25	Washim	-	-	559	68		
				(0.44)	(0.50)		
26	Amravati	2672	285	4553	337	70.4	18.25
		(4.44)	(3.40)	(3.57)	(2.47)		
27	Yavatmal	1196	139	821	120	-31.35	-13.67
		(1.99)	(1.66)	(0.64	(0.88)		

Amravati		6556 (10.9)	706 (8.43)	8940 (7.01)	922 (6.77)	36.36	30.59
28	Wardha	828 (1.38)	89 (1.06)	592 (0.46)	89 (0.65)	-28.5	0.00
29	Nagpur	784 (1.30)	65 (0.78)	1349 (1.06)	105 (0.77)	72.06	61.54
30	Bhandara	271 (0.45)	16 (0.19)	36 (0.03)	4 (0.03)	-86.71	-75.00
31	Gondia	-	-	62 (0.05)	8 (0.06)		
32	Chandrapur	59 (0.10)	8 (0.10)	29 (0.02)	1 (0.01)	-50.85	87.50
33	Gadchiroli	13 (0.02)	1 (0.01)	3 (0.01)	-	-76.92	
Nagpur		1955 (3.25)	179 (2.14	2071 (1.63	207 (1.52	5.93	15.64
Demonstration		(0.79)	476 (3.79)	317	-	-	
Maharashtra		60130 (100.00)	8372 (100.00)	127453 (100.00)	13622 (100.00)	111.96	62.71

Source : Narayanamoorthy, 1996 and Commissionerate of Agriculture, Pune.

Table 2.4
District-wise Area (ha.) Covered and Sets (no.) Distributed of Sprinkler

S.N.	District	2000-01		2001-02		2002-03		2003-04	
		Area	Sets	Area	Sets	Area	Sets	Area	Sets
1	Thane	199.7 (1.33)	216 (1.35)	57.04 (0.73)	55 (0.68)	-	-	4.79 (0.06)	5 (0.06)
2	Raigad	-	-	5.03 (0.06)	8 (0.10)	-	-	-	-
3	Ratnagiri	-	-	11.98 (0.16	24 (0.29	-	-	-	-
4	Sindhudurg	18.91 (0.13)	27 (0.17)	-	-	-	-	1.88 (0.02)	2 (0.02)
Konkan		218.61 (1.46)	243 (1.52)	74.05 (0.95)	87 (1.07)	-	-	6.67 (0.08)	7 (0.08)
5	Nashik	179.88 (1.20)	188 (1.17)	251.6 (3.24)	250 (3.08)	665.01 (5.15)	678 (5.02)	128.7 (1.65)	129 (1.61)
6	Dhule	15.76 (0.11)	15 (0.10)	2 (0.02)	2 (0.02)	60.75 (0.47)	60 (0.44)	8.93 (0.11)	8 (0.10)
7	Nandurbar	5 (0.03)	5 (0.03)	-	-	14 (0.11)	13 (0.10)	4 (0.05)	4 (0.05)
8	Jalgaon	38.51 (0.26)	38 (0.23)	-	-	310.14 (2.40)	319 (2.36)	135.93 (1.75)	132 (1.65)
Nashik		239.15 (1.60)	246 (1.53)	253.6 (3.26)	252 (3.10)	1049.9 (8.13)	1070 (7.92)	277.56 (3.56)	273 (3.41)

9	Ahmednagar	354.24 (2.37)	360 (2.24)	603.69 (7.77)	663 (8.16)	1040.76 (8.06)	1175 (8.69)	1012.13 (13.00)	1117 (13.94)
10	Pune	65 (0.43)	65 (0.41)	154.77 (2.00)	155 (1.91)	23.5 (0.18)	24 (0.18)	174.5 (2.24)	175 (2.19)
11	Solapur	40.15 (0.27)	38 (0.24)	-	-	39 (0.30)	39 (0.29)	120.75 (1.55)	118 (1.47)
Pune		459.39 (3.07)	463 (2.89)	758.46 (9.77)	818 (10.07)	1103.26 (8.54)	1238 (9.16	1307.38 (16.79)	1410 (17.60)
12	Satara	18.13 (0.12)	16 (0.10)	367.52 (4.73)	477 (5.87)	929.51 (7.20)	1160 (8.58)	105.14 (1.35)	105 (1.31)
13	Sangli	36 (0.24)	36 (0.22)	258.91 (3.33)	249 (3.06)	427.96 (3.32)	530 (3.92)	639.4 (8.21)	755 (9.42)
14	Kolhapur	107.5 (0.72)	110 (0.69)	155 (2.00)	156 (1.92)	14 (0.11)	14 (0.10)	101.95 (1.31)	92 (1.15)
Kolhapur		161.63 (1.08)	162 (1.01)	781.43 (10.06)	882 (10.85)	1371.47 (10.63)	1704 (12.60)	846.49 (10.87)	952 (11.88)
15	Aurangabad	25 (0.17)	25 (0.16)	157 (2.02)	157 (1.93)	107 (0.83)	107 (0.79)	78 (1.00)	78 (0.98)
16	Jalna	197 (1.31)	195 (1.21)	33 (0.43)	33 (0.41)	66.9 (0.52)	63 (0.47)	45.27 (0.58)	40 (0.50)
17	Beed	4.55 (0.03)	5 (0.03)	223.09 (2.87)	229 (2.82)	74.78 (0.58)	NA	270.67 (3.48)	271 (3.38)
Aurangabad		226.55 (1.51)	225 (1.40)	413.09 (5.32)	419 (5.16)	248.68 (1.93)	170 (1.26)	393.94 (5.06)	389 (4.86)
18	Latur	852 (5.69)	848 (5.28)	977 (12.58)	977 (12.02)	320 (2.48)	363 (2.69)	346 (4.44)	346 (4.32)

S.N.	District	2000-01		2001-02		2002-03		2003-04	
		Area	Sets	Area	Sets	Area	Sets	Area	Sets
19	Osmanabad	202 (1.35)	202 (1.26)	14 (0.18)	14 (0.17)	163.87 (1.27)	NA	154.6 (1.98)	156 (1.95)
20	Nanded	642.39 (4.29)	646 (4.03)	190.52 (2.45)	191 (2.35)	510 (3.95)	510 (3.95)	566.44 (7.27)	569 (7.10)
21	Hingoli	59 (0.39)	59 (0.37)	127 (1.64)	127 (1.56)	117 (0.91)	117 (0.87)	199.46 (2.56)	204 (2.54)
22	Parbhani	-	-	34.25 (0.44)	35 (0.43)	168 (1.30)	168 (1.24)	130.47 (1.68)	132 (1.65)
Latur		1755.39 (11.72)	1755 (10.94)	1342.77 (17.29)	1344 (16.54)	1278.87 (9.91)	1158 (8.57)	1396.97 (17.93)	1407 (17.56)
23	Buldhana	2179.21 (14.55)	3092 (19.27)	518.1 (6.67)	677 (8.33)	2720.59 (21.08)	2999 (22.19)	624.61 (8.02)	609 (7.60)
24	Akola	2142.06 (14.31)	2150 (13.40)	79 (1.01)	79 (0.97)	665 (5.15)	665 (4.92)	291 (3.73)	278 (3.47)
25	Washim	616.99 (4.12)	698 (4.35)	418.06 (5.38)	384 (4.73)	411.41 (3.19)	439 (3.25)	240.66 (3.09)	255 (3.18)
26	Amravati	1858 (12.41)	1861 (11.60)	368 (4.74)	368 (4.53)	1247.64 (9.67)	1251 (9.26)	584.9 (7.51)	590 (7.37)
27	Yavatmal	2919 (19.50)	2919 (18.20)	557.5 (7.18)	358 (4.40)	904 (7.00)	903 (6.68)	796 (10.22)	797 (9.95)
Amravati		9715.26 (64.89)	10720 (66.82)	1940.66 (24.98)	1866 (22.96)	5948.64 (46.09)	6257 (46.30)	2537.17 (32.57)	2529 (31.57)

28	Wardha	694.31	687	996.63	1243	1114.4	1116	289.12	307
		(4.64)	(4.28)	(12.83)	(15.30)	(8.64)	(8.26)	(3.71)	(3.83)
29	Nagpur	843	843	670	670	409.5	410	468.45	469
		(5.63)	(5.26)	(8.63)	(8.24)	(3.17)	(3.03)	(6.01)	(5.85)
30	Bhandara	171.5	182	74	78	10.5	11	108.81	111
		(1.14)	(1.13)	(0.95)	(0.96)	(0.08)	(0.08)	(1.40)	(1.39)
31	Gondia	132.5	158	8	12	63	69	27.5	28
		(0.88)	(0.98)	(0.10)	(0.15)	(0.49)	(0.51)	(0.35)	(0.35)
32	Chandrapur	332	335	401	402	273.73	274	105	105
		(2.22)	(2.09)	(5.16)	(4.95)	(2.12)	(2.03)	(1.35)	(1.31)
33	Gadchiroli	23.68	24	53.75	53	35	38	24.5	25
		(0.16)	(0.15)	(0.70)	(0.65)	(0.27)	(0.28)	(0.32)	(0.31)
Nagpur		2196.99	2229	2203.38	2458	1906.13	1918	1023.38	1045
		(14.67)	(13.89)	(28.37)	(30.25)	(14.77)	(14.19)	(13.14)	(13.04)
Maharashtra		14973	16043	7767.44	8126	12907	13515	7789.56	8012
		(100.00)	(100.00)	(100.00)	(100.00)	(100.00)	(100.00)	(100.00)	(100.00)

Source : Commissionerate of Agriculture, Pune.

in both areas under and number of sprinkler sets in 2003-04 as compared to 2000-01. But, other divisions (Konkan, Latur, Amravati, and Nagpur) reported negative trend in area and in number of sets during the same period.

2.5 Physical and Financial Achievements of MIS in Study Districts

Physical and financial performance of drip and sprinkler irrigation system over a period of 5 years (2000-01 to 2004-05) in Latur and Osmanabad districts are depicted in Table 2.5. During 2000-01, 216.38 ha. in Latur and 726.34 ha. in Osmanabad district was covered under drip irrigation. In the same fashion, Rs. 40.12 lakhs and Rs. 178.14 lakhs was distributed as subsidy in these two districts. As compared to 2000-01, the area covered under drip and subsidy disbursed during 2004-05 was found 34.6 ha. and Rs. 3.06 lakhs in Latur and 75.80 ha. and Rs. 5.38 lakhs in Osmanabad district respectively. In case of number of sprinkler sets disbursed during 2000-01 were worked out to be 513 and 202 in Latur and Osmanabad respectively. In the same period the amount of subsidy disbursed was Rs. 46.17 lakhs and Rs. 23.29 lakhs in these two districts. During 2004-05, 43 sets of sprinkler irrigation system and Rs. 2.58 lakhs subsidy was disbursed in Latur district, on the other hand in Osmanabad district 5 sets and Rs. 0.21 lakhs subsidy was disbursed. During a period of 5 years, the total area covered under drip and total amount of subsidy disbursed in Latur district was 1365.63 ha. and Rs. 198.09 lakhs at the same time in Osmanabad, 5070.02 ha. of land was covered and Rs. 960.37 lakhs was disbursed as subsidy. In case of sprinkler irrigation system, 2242 sets and Rs. 231.44 lakhs subsidy in Latur district and 528 sets and Rs. 51.76 lakhs subsidy was disbursed in Osmanabad district.

On the whole the area covered as well as subsidy disbursed under drip system in Osmanabad district was more than that of Latur district. On the contrary, number of

Table 2.5
Physical and Financial Achievements of MIS in Study Districts, 2001-05

S.N.	Year	Latur				Osmanabad			
		Drip		Sprinkler		Drip		Sprinkler	
		Phy (ha)	Fin (lakh)	Phy (sets)	Fin (lakh)	Phy (ha)	Fin (lakh)	Phy (sets)	Fin (lakh)
1	2000-01	216.38	40.12	513	46.17	726.34	178.14	202	23.29
2	2001-02	766.79	110.92	977	124.03	416.26	76.51	2	0.24
3	2002-03	38.45	21.24	363	37.9	3625.61	679.19	163	19.26
4	2003-04	309.95	22.75	346	20.76	226.01	21.15	156	8.76
5	2004-05	34.06	3.06	43	2.58	75.8	5.38	5	0.21
	Total	1365.6	198.09	2242	231.44	5070	960.37	528	51.76

Source: Dy. Director (Irrigation), Commissionerate of Agriculture, GoM, Pune.

sprinkler sets and subsidy to sprinkler system disbursed was more in Latur district as compared to Osmanabad district.

2.6 Summary

This chapter deals with growth of MIS in Maharashtra state as well as two selected districts. This chapter also covers physical and financial progress of MIS. In India, Maharashtra state alone accounted for nearly 50% of total drip irrigated area. Area under drip irrigation in Maharashtra has consistently increased from 237 ha. in 1987 to 36958 ha. in 2005, implying a rise of 156 times during the 18 years period. But, development of drip is not uniform across the districts. Total area of drip irrigation under state and central schemes together was 60130 ha. and 127453 ha. during 1986-95 and 2000-05 respectively. In the same fashion, the amount of subsidy disbursed was Rs. 8372 lakhs and Rs. 13622 lakhs respectively. Though, Maharashtra accounts for over 50% of India's total drip irrigated area as of today, its share in sprinkler irrigation comes to only about 5%. During 2000-05, total area covered under drip and total amount of subsidy disbursed in Latur district was 1365.63 ha. and Rs. 198.09 lakhs and that for Osmanabad district it were 5070.02 ha. and Rs. 960.37 lakhs. In case of sprinkler irrigation system, 2242 sets and Rs. 231.44 lakhs subsidy in Latur district and 528 sets and Rs. 51.76 lakhs subsidy was disbursed in Osmanabad district.

On the whole, the area covered as well as subsidy disbursed under drip system in Osmanabad district was more than that of Latur district. On the contrary, number of sprinkler sets and subsidy to sprinkler system disbursed was more in Latur as compared to Osmanabad.

3
Performance of Micro-irrigation System at Farmer's Level

An attempt has been made in this chapter to present the results obtained from field level data, followed by detailed discussion to draw inferences and conclusions against the laid objectives. The results and discussions pertinent to the study are centred around socio-agro-economic characteristics, cropping pattern, factor motivating farmers to adopt drip/ sprinkler, and cost of cultivation for different crops vis-à-vis comparative economics and productivity enhancement due to adoption of drip/sprinkler technology. Besides that an attempt was also made to ascertain the minimization of yield and price uncertainties before and after adoption of MIS in selected crops. Further, efforts also made to assess the capital and production cost with respect to subsidy administration aspects. Accordingly, arrived results are discussed and provided in following sections.

3.1 Profiles of Sample Farmers

Socio-agro-economic characteristics influence cropping pattern, resource use, decision making, etc. The characteristics, viz.: age, education, sex, family size, social group, land holding, annual income, and farming experience were examined in the study area and the observations are presented in Table 3.1.

The table reveals that about 41% drip adopters were more than 50 years and 44% sprinkler adopters were in the age group of 31-40 years at overall level. Across districts, the majority of drip and sprinkler adopters in Latur district were found in the age group of more than 50 years. Compared to Osmanabad district, drip and sprinkler adopters of Latur district are in the age group of more energetic and risk-taking category. As regards formal schooling, about 57% drip adopters and 61% sprinkler adopters had up to HSC level education followed by graduate and higher level of education and worked out to the tune of 25% and 24% respectively at overall level. Considering a vital role of education in judicious decision-making, technology adoption, and bringing in transformation; educational base of sample farmers is found satisfactory. Further, despite special subsidy incentive for ladies by Government of Maharashtra only 18% of drip and 30% of sprinkler female adopters reported in the study area indicates slow pace of MIS adoption among ladies category. Accordingly, there is scope for further awareness and MIS adoption among women. Social group-wise analysis depicts disproportionate picture as the majority of drip and sprinkler adopters belonged to general category (55% and 69% respectively) followed by OBC category (28% and 14% respectively). Comparatively SC (13% and 8% respectively) and ST (4% and 8% respectively) categories had lower representation and hence scope. Present land ceiling act of the state government and disintegration of joint families resulted in diminishing size of land-holdings. On the other hand, present cropping pattern, capital cost of drip/sprinkler, and farming experience imposes constraints in MIS adoption. Accordingly, majority of drip and sprinkler adopters were found in medium (5 to 20 acres) and large (>20 acres) land holding categories having more than 3 lakhs annual income

Table 3.1
District-wise Socio-agro-economic Characteristics of Sample Farmers

S.N.	Characteristics	Category	Latur			
			Drip (n=136)		Sprinkler (n=224)	
			No.	%	No.	%
1	Age (years)	< 30	9	6.62	7	3.13
		31- 40	64	47.06	109	48.66
		41 – 50	35	25.73	36	16.07
		> 50	28	20.59	72	32.14
2	Education	Illiterate	13	9.56	36	16.07
		HSC	93	68.38	130	58.04
		Graduate & more	30	22.06	58	25.89
3	Sex	Male	106	77.94	152	67.86
		Female	30	22.06	72	32.14
4	Family size	< 5	25	18.38	22	9.82
		5-8	42	30.88	115	51.34
		> 8	69	50.74	87	38.84
5	Social group	SC	13	9.56	14	6.25
		ST	4	2.94	21	9.37

		OBC	47	34.56	29	12.95
		General	72	52.94	160	71.43
6	Land holding (acres)	Small (< 5)	21	15.44	28	12.50
		Medium (5.1-20)	76	55.88	145	64.73
		Large (> 20)	39	28.68	51	22.77
7	Annual income (Rs.)	< 1 lakhs	21	15.44	57	25.45
		1-3 lakhs	42	30.88	73	32.59
		> 3 lakhs	73	53.68	94	41.96
8	Farming experience (years)	< 5	4	2.94	-	-
		5-10	21	15.44	29	12.95
		> 10	111	81.62	195	87.05

Table 3.1: contd…

S.N.	Characteristics		Osmanabad				Total			
			Drip (n=507)		Sprinkler (n=53)		Drip (n=643)		Sprinkler (n=277)	
			No.	%	No.	%	No.	%	No.	%
1	Age (years)	< 30	34	6.61	4	7.55	43	6.69	11	3.97
		31- 40	135	26.63	12	22.64	199	30.95	121	43.68
		41 – 50	101	19.92	9	16.98	136	21.15	45	16.25
		> 50	237	46.74	28	52.83	265	41.21	100	36.10
2	Education	Illiterate	102	20.12	6	9.43	115	17.88	42	15.16
		HSC	276	54.24	39	73.58	369	57.39	169	61.01
		Graduate & more	129	25.44	8	15.10	159	24.73	66	23.83
3	Sex	Male	422	83.23	42	79.25	528	82.12	194	70.04
		Female	85	16.77	11	20.75	115	17.88	83	29.96
4	Family size	< 5	99	19.53	5	9.43	124	19.28	27	9.75
		5-8	247	48.72	35	66.04	289	44.95	150	54.15
		> 8	161	31.75	13	24.53	230	35.77	100	36.10
5	Social group	SC	68	13.41	9	16.98	81	12.60	23	8.30
		ST	24	4.73	2	3.77	28	4.35	23	8.30

		OBC	133	26.24	10	18.87	180	28.00	39	14.08
		General	282	55.62	32	60.38	354	55.05	192	69.32
6	Land holding (acres)	Small (< 5)	63	12.43	13	24.53	84	13.06	41	14.80
		Medium (5.1-20)	355	70.02	34	64.15	431	67.03	179	64.62
		Large (> 20)	89	17.55	6	11.32	128	19.91	57	20.58
7	Annual income (Rs.)	< 1 lakhs	118	23.27	24	45.28	139	21.62	81	29.24
		1-3 lakhs	203	40.04	16	30.19	245	38.10	89	32.13
		> 3 lakhs	186	36.69	13	24.53	259	40.28	107	38.63
8	Farming experience (years)	< 5	51	10.06	4	7.55	55	8.55	4	1.44
		5-10	118	23.27	16	30.19	139	21.62	45	16.25
		>10	338	66.67	33	62.26	449	69.83	228	82.31

Source : Field study.

and better (>10 years) farming experience. Across districts, with little exception, similar trend was observed.

From above observations it could be concluded that majority of sample drip/sprinkler adopters were better educated males of general category having better experience in farming with medium to large land holdings and satisfactory annual income.

3.2 Land Holding

Information regarding cultivated, uncultivated land, and area under drip and sprinkler irrigation of sample farmers from Latur and Osmanabad district is given in Table 3.2.

It can be observed from the table that at overall level proportion of irrigated land to total land holding was quite high (67%). Further, area under drip irrigation was found on higher side (37%) compared to sprinkler irrigation (17%). District-wise scenario also revealed the high proportion (>60%) of irrigated land among both the districts. However, individual coverage of sprinkler irrigation was found more (33%) in Latur district and that for drip irrigation (53%) in Osmanabad district. Further, proportion of area under dry farming (22%) and uncultivated land (12%) at overall level indicate scope for further expansion of MIS.

3.3 Cropping Pattern

Existing agro-climatic conditions, soil type, and availability of water determines the cropping pattern of any area. In this context, an attempt has been made to study the irrigation-wise cropping pattern of study area. Results are provided in Table 3.3.

It could be observed from the table that individual irrigation method-wise area under sprinkler in Latur district contributed highest (37%) share to the total cultivated land followed by dry (27%), drip (22%), and surface (14%) method of irrigation. While that for Osmanabad district it was drip

Table 3.2
District-wise Landholding (acres) Details

S.N.	District	Cultivated		Uncultivated	Total	Area under	
		Irrigated	Dry			Drip	Sprinkler
1	Latur	4278.64 (64.18)	1615.07 (24.22)	773.07 (11.60)	6666.78 (100.00)	1272.96 (19.10)	2186.38 (32.80)
2	Osmanabad	5484.16 (68.51)	1566.36 (19.57)	954.5 (11.92)	8005.02 (100.00)	4215.93 (52.67)	367.37 (4.59)
3	Total	9762.8 (66.54)	3181.43 (21.68)	1727.57 (11.78)	14671.8 (100.00)	5488.89 (37.41)	2553.75 (17.41)

Figures in brackets indicate percentage to total.
Source : Field study.

Table 3.3
District-wise Cropping Pattern (acres)

S.N.	District	Crop	Irrigated			Dry	Total
			Drip	Sprinkler	Surface		
1	Latur	Sugarcane	623.33 (48.97)	895.27 (40.95)	293.87 (35.87)	-	1812.47 (30.75)
		Grapes	411.46 (32.32)	-	162.32 (19.81)	-	573.78 (9.74)
		Cereal	-	311.57	57.72	994.03	1363.32

				(14.25)	(7.04)	(61.55)	(23.13)
		Pulses	-	665.27	154.74	393.48	1213.49
				(30.43)	(18.89)	(24.36)	(20.59)
		Oilseeds	-	120.88	94.2	153.82	368.9
				(5.53)	(11.50)	(9.52)	(6.26)
		Others	238.17	193.39	56.45	73.74	561.75
			(18.71)	(8.84)	(6.89)	(4.57)	(9.53)
		Total	1272.96	2186.38	819.3	1615.07	5893.71
			(21.60)	(37.10)	(13.90)	(27.40)	(100.00)
2	Osmanabad	Sugarcane	2574.21	90.51	255.48	-	2920.2
			(61.06)	(24.64)	(28.36)		(41.42)
		Grapes	978.56	-	131.35	-	1109.91
			(23.21)		(14.58)		(15.74)
		Cereal	-	81.75	110.13	762.97	954.85
				(22.25)	(12.22)	(48.71)	(13.55)
		Pulses	-	160.51	223.66	366.21	750.38
				(43.69)	(24.83)	(23.38)	(10.64)
		Oilseeds	-	21.93	116.5	254.38	392.81
				(5.97)	(12.93)	(16.24)	(5.57)
		Others	663.16	12.67	63.74	182.8	922.37
			(15.73)	(3.45)	(7.08)	(11.67)	(13.08)
		Total	4215.93	367.37	900.86	1566.36	7050.52
			(59.80)	(5.21)	(12.78)	(22.21)	(100.00)

Figures in brackets indicate percentage to total.
Source : Field study.

(60%) followed by dry (22%), surface (13%), and sprinkler (5%) method of irrigation.

Further, crop-wise cropping pattern analysis revealed the dominance of sugarcane in total cultivated land of Latur (31%) and Osmanabad (41%) district followed by cereal (23%), pulses (21%), and grapes (10%) in Latur district and grapes (16%), cereal (14%), and 'others' (13%) in Osmanabad district. 'Others' category included crops like vegetables, mango, ber, pomegranate, etc.

Across districts, crops and individual method of irrigation, sugarcane under drip contributed highest (61%) share in Osmanabad district followed by grapes (32%) in Latur district. Further, pulses under sprinkler shared highest (44%) share in Osmanabad district followed by sugarcane (41%), and pulses (30%) in Latur district. Traditional surface method of irrigation mainly practiced for sugarcane (36% in Latur and 28% in Osmanabad district), and grapes (20% in Latur district). Commercially not so important cereals (61% in Latur district and 49% in Osmanabad district), and pulses (24% in Latur and 23% in Osmanabad district) were cultivated as rainfed crops.

From above analysis it could be concluded that sprinkler technology is more popular in Latur district and drip technology in Osmanabad district for cultivation of cash crops (sugarcane, grapes, vegetables, fruit crops, etc). While not-so-remunerative food-grains (cereal, pulses, and oilseeds) were cultivated as rainfed crops. However, substantial percentage under surface method of irrigation (14% in Latur and 13% in Osmanabad district), and dry farming (27% in Latur and 22% in Osmanàbad district) warrants need for efficient use of scare water. In this context, there is a wide scope for bringing this area under MIS in both the districts.

3.4 Motivation Factors for Adoption of Drip/Sprinkler Technology

Sample farmers of the study area were interviewed to probe

into the rationale behind adoption of drip/sprinkler technology and the relevant observations are presented in Table 3.4.

It is discernable from the table that the most influencing factors for farmers to adopt drip technology at overall level were prolonged power cuts (89%), followed by less water requirement (80%), subsidy (70%), reduction in cost of cultivation (64%), labour saving (63%), and increase in yield (61%). While that for adoption of sprinkler technology it were increase in yield (84%), prolonged power cuts (75%), less water requirements (68%), and reduction in cost of cultivation (57%).

Across districts and technology, more than 50% sample farmers from Latur district adopt drip technology owing to less water requirement (95%), prolonged power cuts (87%), increase in yield (72%), labour saving (63%), and to reduce weed problem (51%). Interestingly, subsidy factor was not found much appealing for sample farmers of Latur district. Compared to this, sample farmers of Osmanabad district preferred drip technology because of prolonged power cuts (89%), subsidy (81%), less water requirement (76%), reduction in cost of cultivation (68%), labour saving (63%), and increase in yield (58%).

In case of adoption of sprinkler technology by sample farmers of Latur district major influencing factors were found similar in order to that of overall level. However, for Osmanabad district they were prolonged power cuts (81%), less water requirement (78%), reduction in cost of cultivation (72%), increase in yield (66%), and labour saving (58%).

From above results it could be inferred that besides proven fact of water saving ability of drip and sprinkler technology acute power shortage (from 14-18 hours load shedding per day and low voltage supply) forced the sample farmers to adopt these technologies. The rationale behind this was to save their valuable crops from wilting and also to irrigate more area within a limited time period of power

Table 3.4
Factors Motivating Farmers to Adopt Drip/Sprinkler Irrigation

S.N.	Particular		LWR	LS	SBS	ASE	WP	RCC	UT	IY	IQO	FS	ES	PPC
1	Latur													
	Drip	No.	129	86	38	22	70	65	25	98	43	50	29	118
		%	94.85	63.23	27.94	16.18	51.47	47.8	18.38	72.06	31.62	36.76	21.32	86.76
	Sprinkler	No.	148	107	92	27	64	119	82	197	47	38	54	164
		%	66.07	47.76	41.07	12.05	28.57	53.12	36.61	87.95	20.98	16.96	24.11	73.21
2	Osmanabad													
	Drip	No.	387	318	411	105	212	346	67	292	190	159	132	452
		%	76.33	62.72	81.06	20.71	41.81	68.24	13.21	57.6	37.47	31.36	26.03	89.15
	Sprinkler	No.	41	31	24	5	10	38	26	35	19	8	11	43
		%	78.36	58.5	45.28	9.43	18.87	71.7	49.05	66.03	35.85	15.1	20.75	81.13
3	Total													
	Drip	No.	516	404	449	127	282	411	92	390	233	209	161	570
		%	80.25	62.83	69.83	19.75	43.86	63.92	14.31	60.65	36.24	32.5	25.04	88.65
	Sprinkler	No.	189	138	116	32	74	157	108	232	66	46	65	207
		%	68.23	49.82	41.88	11.55	26.71	56.68	38.98	83.75	23.83	16.61	23.46	74.73

Source : Field study.

Note: LWR= Less Water Requirement, LS= Labour saving, SBS= Subsidy, ASE= Avoid Soil Erosion, WP= Weed Problem, RCC= Reduce Cost of Cultivation, UT= Uneven Terrain, IY= Increase Yield, IQO= Improve Quality of Output, FS= Fertilizer Saving, ES= Energy Saving, and PPC= Prolonged Power Cuts.

available compared to traditional surface irrigation method. The analysis also revealed that subsidy factor in drip technology was not much attractive for farmers of Latur district despite a high capital cost. This is against the popular perception that farmers adopt drip technology because of heavy subsidy. This was because of realization of advantages of drip technology by farmers on one hand and because of insufficient subsidy amount, too much delayed disbursement of subsidy, and mis-handling of subsidy issue by dealers as well as government officers on the other hand. However, farmers of Osmanabad district strongly accepted the subsidy influence. Further, subsidy component in sprinkler technology was not found much appealing in either of the districts because of low capital cost and hence within the reach of willing farmers.

Drip technology definitely helps in weed minimization and hence in labour saving through reducing intercultural operations and also by by-passing the practice of manning the conveyance channel while irrigating by traditional method of irrigation. Accordingly, factors like labour saving and reduction in cost of cultivation were duely reflected in farmers' opinion. However, factors like fertilizer saving and energy saving did not appear as per the expectation. Because of costly liquid fertilizers and fear of chocking drippers general tendency of farmers is to avoid fertigation and to save fertilizers by method of avoiding wastage. Further, because of prolonged power cuts they are tempted to utilize the electricity as long as available (6-10 hours/day).

In case of sprinkler besides water saving and power cuts, increase in yield emerged as important influencing factor. This was because of multi-utility of sprinkler technology like convenience in physical movement, applicability over uneven terrain, and suitability for closed space crops like vegetables, cereals, pulses, oilseed, and even in sugarcane at early stage. While on the other hand, above mentioned crops though generally cultivated as rainfed, 2 to 3 protective irrigations at critical stages are useful to avoid water stress and hence ultimately resulted in increased in yield compared to rainfed conditions. Hence, besides low capital cost and maintenance cost, factors mentioned above added popularity to sprinkler among sample farmers.

3.5 Technical Awareness about MIS

In a given scenario of standard guidelines laid down by Government of Maharashtra for manufacturers, dealers, government officers, and beneficiary farmers an attempt has been made to know the awareness of sample farmers about select parameters and results are provided in Table 3.5.

Farmers receive information related to new technology in agriculture from various sources. Government extension officers have important role in disseminating such information. However, study results revealed that sample farmers at overall level mostly contacted dealers (30%) to solve their problems (Table 3.5). Sugar factories operating in study area, relatives, etc., clubbed together as 'others' were the second most (28%) source of information for farmers followed by co-villagers (21%), and government officers (19%). Further, district-wise analysis revealed that once again dealers (33%) were the important source of information in Latur district followed by government officer (27%), and co-villagers (24%). However, for Osmanabad district 'others' were the major (36%) source of information followed by dealers (19%), and government officers (14%). Special drive was under taken by Terna Sugar Factory (TSF) for drip promotion in its jurisdiction in Osmanabad district. For that purpose besides government's 75% subsidy on drip set, TSF promised additional 15% subsidy (thus amounting to 90% subsidy) for their member-farmers. This was the principal reason behind mass awareness as well as adoption of drip technology in Osmanabad district. Accordingly, sample farmers of Osmanabad district mainly adopted this technology during 2002-03 (44%) followed by 2001-02 (22%), and 2000-01 (16%).

Compared to this the technology adoption rate among Latur district was found highest (35%) in 2000-01 followed by 2003-04 (24%), and 2001-02 (17%). However, the technology adoption rate among both the districts was found inconsistent during the period under consideration.

Farmers willing to avail subsidy for drip/sprinkler are supposed to prepare and submit the proposal to Taluka Agriculture Officer (TAO) by themselves. However, owing to lack of information about the procedure, documents required, physical distance to be covered, time and other constraints sample farmers preferred dealer, who in turn get assured customers, perform this job for his customer-farmers. About 60% farmer's proposal in Latur district and 46% in Osmanabad district were prepared and submitted by dealers followed by 'others' including sugar factory, co-villager, relatives, etc. (19% and 34% in Latur and Osmanabad district respectively). Further, majority (64% and 72% in Latur and Osmanabad district respectively) of farmers received acknowledgment for their submitted proposals.

As per the government's guideline manufacturer and dealers of drip/sprinkler are compelled to supply only BIS quality materials. However, owing to farmers' unawareness about such technical aspects, probability of cheating arises. Accordingly, sample farmers were asked for self-verification of such BIS/embossed quality marks. Unfortunately, more than 60% farmers from both the districts did not verify such quality assurance marks themselves. Hence, training and awareness efforts for self-verification of such quality marks are in order. Regarding the laid norms of warranty period for drip/sprinkle set, majority (97% and 77% in Latur and Osmanabad districts respectively) of farmers reported affirmative. However, 23% farmers from Osmanabad districts were denied to avail this facility.

Technically correct irrigation layout/design has paramount importance in success of MIS from efficiency and durable working point of view. Such design, however, depends on

Table 3.5
Technical Awareness of Farmers about MIS

S.N.	Particulars	Category	Latur (n=360)		Osmanabad (n=560)		Total (n=920)	
			No.	%	No.	%	No.	%
1	Source of information	a) Govt. agency	97	26.94	78	13.93	175	19.02
		b) Dealer	120	33.33	158	28.21	278	30.22
		c) Co-villagers	86	23.89	109	19.46	195	21.19
		d) Media	6	1.67	11	1.97	17	1.85
		e) Others	51	14.17	204	36.43	255	27.72
2	Year of adoption	a) 2000-01	126	35	90	16.07	216	23.48
		b) 2001-02	62	17.22	123	21.96	185	20.11
		c) 2002-03	45	12.5	246	43.93	291	31.63
		d) 2003-04	87	24.17	67	11.97	154	16.74
		e) 2004-05	40	11.11	34	6.07	74	8.04
3	Preparation and submission of proposal	a) Self	23	6.39	46	8.21	69	7.5
		b) Dealer	217	60.28	257	45.9	474	51.52
		c) Govt. officer	51	14.17	66	11.78	117	12.72
		d) Others	69	19.16	191	34.11	260	28.26
4	Acknowledgement for submitted proposal	a) Yes	229	63.61	403	71.96	632	68.7
		b) No	131	36.39	157	28.04	288	31.3

5	Awareness about bank loan for drip/sprinkler	a) Yes	303	84.17	447	79.82	750	81.52
		b) No	57	15.83	113	20.18	170	18.48
6	Self verification of BIS mark or embossing on received set	a) Yes	126	35	213	38.04	339	36.85
		b) No	234	65	347	61.96	581	63.15
7	Warranty period	a) Yes	348	96.67	432	77.14	780	84.78
		b) No	12	3.33	128	22.86	140	15.22
8	Irrigation layout designed by	a) Self	24	6.67	33	5.9	57	6.2
		b) Dealer	320	88.89	482	86.07	802	87.17
		c) Others	16	4.44	45	8.03	61	6.63

Source : Field study.

number of factors like crop to be irrigated, spacing adopted, soil type, quality, source and availability of water, temperature, etc., and hence needs great caution while designing and laying. Obviously with a poor technical knowledge majority (>86%) of sample farmers from both the districts depends on the technical services (Agricultural Engineer) of dealer for designing and laying the irrigation layout. Carelessness and error on the part of dealer/engineer greatly affects the interest of beneficiary-farmers. Hence, farmers training and assistance of government agencies are in order.

3.6 Investment Pattern in Drip and Sprinkler

One of the arguments for the less adoption of drip and sprinkler technology is about their capital intensive nature, especially in case of drip technology. Accordingly, subsidies by government and loans by banks are being provided to the farmers who are ready to adopt these technologies. In this context an attempt was made to understand investment pattern in drip and sprinkler in the study districts. The observations are presented in Table 3.6.

Individual technology-wise investment pattern revealed that per acre average investment made by sample farmers in drip varied from Rs. 53045 (<5 acres category) to Rs. 41776 (>20 acres category) at overall level. While that for sprinkler it ranged between Rs. 20315 (<5 acres category) to Rs. 18625 (>20 acres category). Thus, negative correlation was reported between size of land holding and average investment made in drip/sprinkler. This was because of economies of scale achieved by big farmers.

Source-wise investment pattern at overall level revealed that comparatively sprinkler adopters invested more of own funds over bank loans than drip adopters. Being capital intensive, investments made in drip by sample farmers are substantially supported by bank loans. However, against the prevailing 50% subsidy norm, maximum subsidy availed by sample farmers was reported to the tune of 32% in drip and 37% in sprinkler in both the districts by the farmers having 5-20 acres land. This was because of company-wise different rates of drip/sprinkler set, crops cultivated, spacing adopted, type of irrigation layout, distance from source of water, etc. Accordingly, actual cost per set of drip/sprinkler in the study area was found always on higher side than the prescribed cost by government and hence percentage of subsidy to total capital cost appeared less. In this context 50% subsidy provision of total capital cost compared to actual market price not realized in practical. Hence, feelings of farmers on this issue are very strong. In this context, government should handle this issue in more realistic manner based on actual market-price. Further, necessary policy amendments are in order.

Across districts and technology, average investment pattern was found highest (Rs. 55538) in case of drip in Osmanabad district and that for Rs. 21344 in case of sprinkler in Latur district. Besides above mentioned cost escalating factors, drip adoption by sample farmers of Osmanabad district was comparatively late and hence drip set cost them more. Further, except sprinkler adopters of Osmanabad district, negative correlation was observed between size of land holdings and investment made in drip/sprinkler in both the districts. Percentage of subsidy to the total capital cost in case of drip adopters of Latur district was found on higher side compared to Osmanabad district. However, maximum percentage of subsidy availed by sample drip adopters of Latur district was reported to 36% in > 20 acres land holding category while that for Osmanabad district it was 30% in the same category. The maximum (39%) percentage of subsidy availed by sample sprinkler adopters was found in Osmanabad district compared to 36% in Latur district.

Sample farmers of Latur district invested more of own capital compared to their counterparts in Osmanabad district to meet the total capital requirement of drip/sprinkler.

Table 3.6
Per Household Average Investment Pattern (Rs.) of Drip/Sprinkler Farmers

S.N.	District	MIS	Category	Source of Investment			Total
				Bank	Own	Subsidy	
1	Latur	Drip	< 5 acres	-	31697 (69.56)	13871 (30.44)	45568 (100.00)
			5-20 acres	-	29529 (66.60)	14810 (33.40)	44339 (100.00)
			> 20 acres	6054 (14.14)	21492 (50.19)	15274 (35.67)	42820 (100.00)
		Sprinkler	< 5 acres	-	14261 (66.82)	7083 (33.18)	21344 (100.00)
			5(20 acres	-	12210 (63.90)	6899 (36.10)	19109 (100.00)
			> 20 acres	1002 (5.40)	11529 (62.17)	6015 (32.43)	18546 (100.00)
2	Osmanabad	Drip	< 5 acres	20792 (37.44)	20507 (36.92)	14239 (25.64)	55538 (100.00)
			5-20 acres	27451 (50.33)	14886 (27.29)	12205 (22.38)	54542 (100.00)
			> 20 acres	12377 (29.95)	16367 (39.61)	12576 (30.44)	41320 (100.00)
		Sprinkler	< 5 acres	2343 (12.95)	10504 (58.04)	5250 (29.01)	18097 (100.00)
			5-20 acres	1636	11054	7991	20681

				(7.91)	(53.45)	(38.64)	(100.00)
			> 20 acres	-	12406	6892	19298
					(64.29)	(35.71)	(100.00)
3	Total	Drip	< 5 acres	15594	23304	14147	53045
				(29.40)	(43.93)	(26.67)	(100.00)
			5-20 acres	22610	17468	12664	52742
				(42.87)	(33.12)	(24.01)	(100.00)
			> 20 acres	10450	17928	13398	41776
				(25.02)	(42.91)	(32.07)	(100.00)
		Sprinkler	< 5 acres	743	13070	6502	20315
				(3.66)	(64.34)	(32.00)	(100.00)
			5-20 acres	311	11990	7106	19407
				(1.60)	(61.78)	(36.62)	(100.00)
			> 20 acres	897	11621	6107	18625
				(4.82)	(62.39)	(32.79)	(100.00)

Figures in brackets indicate percentage to total.
Source : Field study.

Comparatively more bank loan in case of Osmanabad district was because of TSF's policy. In the wake of late subsidy disbursement from government, TSF too not kept its commitment for additional 15% subsidy. Further, without consulting member-farmers TSF converted their capital expenditure into bank loans and started recovery from their cane-payment and served notice for their land-seizing. Owing to these unpleasant developments farmers feel cheated and want justice.

3.7 Non-functioning of Installed Sets

Dis-functioning of installed MI sets is either temporary or permanent. Temporary disfunctioning of drip sets is mainly because of clogging of drippers owing to salt deposition, fungal growth, and plant roots. Rat bites and mud formation during rainy season also leads to temporary disfunctioning of drip sets. While permanent disfunctioning of drip sets is mainly because of sub-standard quality of supplied sets which leads to cracking of laterals. Farmers' ignorance about periodical acid wash of drip sets lead to permanent salt deposition/fungal growth in drippers and hence non-functioning of the sets.

Reasons for temporary disfunctioning of sprinklers are clogging of raisers nozzle, and non-revolving of raiser. While, breakage of pipes owing to sub-standard quality and mis-handling leads to permanent non-functioning of sprinkler set. Besides above mentioned factors frequent load shedding, low voltage supply, rainy season, and non-availability of water during summer leads to temporary non-functioning of MI sets.

Despite the government's guideline for supply of BIS quality materials and specified warranty period for drip/ sprinkler set, some cases of non-functioning of drip/sprinkler sets within 3 to 6 months from installation were noticed in study districts (Table 3.7). In all 11.66% of drip and 14.44% of sprinkler sets were reported as temporarily non-functioning and 21.62% of drip and 6.14% of sprinkler sets were reported as permanently non-functioning in the study area. Across study districts, highest percentages of temporarily non-functioning drip and sprinkler sets were reported in Osmanabad (13.41 and 20.75 respectively). Those for permanently non-functioning drip and sprinkler sets were reported in Osmanabad (26.63%) and Latur (6.25%) district respectively.

Results clearly revealed that across MI technologies and study districts problem of non-functioning of MI sets is major in drip technology adopted by beneficiary-farmers of Osmanabad district. Principal reason is sub-standard quality of drip sets supplied in the district coupled with ignorance of farmers about regular acid wash, and physical impurities in water.

Further, failure of TSF to fulfil additional 15% subsidy, converting capital cost of drip sets in bank loan without the consent of farmers, and notice to seize their lands aggravated the situation in Osmanabad district. This created great unrest among farmers and they sued the Government of Maharashtra, TSF, and Nagarjuna company (manufacturer and supplier of drip set). Presently the matter is subjudice and farmers eagerly waiting for justice. Such a scenario revealed the pathetic picture of the scheme in TSF jurisdiction and hence brought bad name to all concerned including state government. Hence, implementing officers as well as executing officers need to be more alert about physical verification and strict spot assessment to ensure prescribed quality standards. Further, subsidy should be disbursed as quick as possible.

3.8 Cost of Cultivation

As mentioned in Chapter 1 (1.8), cost of cultivation was worked out separately for drip and sprinkler system vis-à-vis traditional method using two crops each (sugarcane and grapes for drip, and sugarcane and gram for sprinkler). Farmers were asked to indicate cost of cultivation in both the

Table 3.7
Non-functioning of Installed Sets

SN	Particulars	Latur (n= 136)		Osmanabad (n= 507)		Total (n= 643)	
		Temporary	Permanent	Temporary	Permanent	Temporary	Permanent
1	Drip	17 (12.50)	4 (2.94)	68 (13.41)	135 (26.63)	75 (11.66)	139 (21.62)
		Latur (n= 224)		Osmanabad (n= 53)		Total (n= 277)	
2	Sprinkler	29 (12.95)	14 (6.25)	11 (20.75)	3 (5.66)	40 (14.44)	17 (6.14)

Figures in brackets indicate percentage to respective total.
Source : Field study.

methods of irrigation (traditional verses improved). In all, 643 drip adopters and 277 sprinkler adopters formed part of the sample. The results are provided in Tables 3.8 to 3.11.

It could be observed from Table 3.8 that in Latur district drip technology in case of sugarcane reduced the total cost of cultivation by Rs. 7476/acre (38%) over traditional method of irrigation. However, percentages of savings vary across different operations. Per acre savings in costs under drip technology in absolute term was found highest for fertilizers (Rs. 2144) followed by labour cost of irrigation (Rs. 1813), seed and sowing (Rs. 891), and electricity charges (Rs. 784). This was mainly because of avoiding wastage and adoption of fertigation, savings of labour in control of water supply, changing course of water, governing leakages and seepages, and ability of drip technology to irrigate larger area in short period of time compared to traditional method of irrigation.

Average per acre cost of sugarcane cultivation under drip technology in Latur district worked out to be Rs. 19429 compared to Rs. 26905 in traditional method (Table 3.8). However, item-wise maximum contribution to the total cost under drip technology was reported in seed and sowing (22%) followed by fertilizers (19%), FYM (18%), and land preparation (17%). That for traditional method it were fertilizers (22%), seed and sowing (19%), FYM (15%), land preparation (14%), and labour cost of irrigation (10%).

Further, it could also be observed from the table that drip technology reduced the total cost of sugarcane cultivation by Rs. 7476/acre (38%) over traditional method in Latur district. However, amount and percentage of saving in terms of rupees was found highest for fertilizers (Rs. 2144) followed by labour cost of irrigation (Rs. 1813), seed and sowing (Rs. 891), and electricity charges (Rs. 784).

Generally, cost of cultivation varies with crops as the nature of operation and input requirement varies. For example, use of pesticide in sugarcane is very low while it is must for grapes. Considering this difference an attempt has been made

Table 3.8
Cost of Cultivation (Rs/acre) for Study crops under Drip in Latur District

S.N.	Item	Sugarcane			Grapes		
		Drip	Traditional	Saving	Drip	Traditional	Saving
1	Land preparation	3257.14 (16.76)	3742.53 (13.91)	485.39 (14.90)	6565.22 (5.50)	7010.35 (4.86)	445.13 (6.78)
2	Seed and sowing	4285.71 (22.06)	5176.66 (19.24)	890.95 (20.79)	9282.61 (7.78)	9326.1 (6.47)	43.49 (0.47)
3	Fertilizer	3785.05 (19.48)	5928.57 (22.03)	2143.52 (56.63)	21678.3 (18.16)	26873.9 (18.63)	5195.65 (23.97)
4	FYM	3571.43 (18.38)	4021.17 (14.95)	449.74 (12.60)	8523.9 (7.14)	8652.17 (6.00)	128.27 (1.50)
5	Pesticide	85.13 (0.44)	142.86 (0.53)	57.73 (67.81)	34176.5 (28.63)	40217.4 (27.89)	6040.87 (17.67)
6	Intercultural operations	1285.58 (6.62)	1857.14 (6.90)	571.56 (44.46)	12331.3 (10.33)	18352.2 (12.73)	6020.86 (48.82)
7	Irrigation a) labour	914.29 (4.71)	2727.68 (10.14)	1813.39 (198.34)	2962.17 (2.48)	8367.39 (5.80)	5405.22 (182.47)
	b) Electricity charges	1501.66 (7.73)	2285.71 (8.50)	784.05 (52.21)	3645.65 (3.05)	6891.3 (4.78)	3245.65 (89.03)
8	Harvesting	-	-	-	9173.91 (7.69)	9369.57 (6.5)	195.66 (2.13)

9	Transportation & mktg.	-	-	-	10043.5 (8.41)	8086.96 (5.61)	(1956.5 (19.48)
10	Others	742.58 (3.82)	1022.43 (3.80)	279.85 (37.68)	991.74 (0.83)	1052.61 (0.73)	60.87 (6.14)
	Total	19428.6 (100.00)	26904.8 (100.00)	7476.18 (38.48)	119375 (100.00)	144200 (100.00)	24825.2 (20.79)

Figures in brackets indicate percentage to total and that for under 'saving' column indicates percentage of corresponding saving.
Source : Field study.

to understand the impact of drip on grapes cultivation in study area.

Table 3.8 further revealed that Rs. 119375/acre was incurred on grapes cultivation under drip technology compared to Rs. 144200/acre under traditional method. Across different items of costs pesticides, fertilizers, and intercultural operations in given order contributed maximum share to total cost for both the categories.

Further, it could be observed from the table that drip technology saved more amounts for grapes (Rs. 24825) than sugarcane (Rs. 7476) on per acre basis in Latur district. However, operation-wise saving in grapes cultivation was found highest in cost of pesticide (Rs. 6041) followed by intercultural operations (Rs. 6021), labour cost of irrigation (Rs. 5405), fertilizers (Rs. 5196), and charges of electricity (Rs. 3246). Contrary to this, because of distant transportations and frequent grading cost incurred on transportation and marketing by drip adopters was found on higher side (Rs. 1957) compared to their counterparts.

Cost of cultivation also varies with the method of irrigation adopted. Accordingly, attempt has been made to study the impact of sprinkler irrigation over traditional method with respect to sugarcane and gram crops in Latur district. Results are presented in Table 3.9.

Per acre average cost of sugarcane cultivation under sprinkler technology worked out to be Rs. 21031 compared to Rs. 25834 under traditional method and hence helped sample farmers to save Rs. 4803 (23%)/acre by adoption of sprinkler technology for sugarcane (Table 3.9). Item-wise percentage share of cost incurred on sugarcane cultivation under sprinkler technology was found highest (24%) for fertilizers followed by seed and sowing (22%), FYM (16%), land preparation (15%), and electricity charges (9%). For traditional method, major items of cost were found in similar order as that of sprinkler technology but with different percentages. However, labour cost for irrigation in case of sugarcane under traditional method was found quite high (Rs. 3025) if compared to its counterpart (Rs. 752). Operation-wise savings in case of sugarcane under sprinkler technology was reported highest for labour cost of irrigation (Rs. 2273) followed by fertilizers (Rs. 688), and intercultural operations (Rs. 673).

Further, per acre average cost of gram cultivation under sprinkler technology in Latur district reported to be Rs. 9982 compared to Rs. 11393 under traditional method. Thus, about Rs. 1411 (14%) could be saved per acre by means of adoption of sprinkler technology. However, item-wise cost incurred on gram cultivation under sprinkler technology revealed the maximum share of seed and sowing (Rs. 1881) followed by fertilizers (Rs. 1625), and FYM (Rs. 1137%). Compared to this, gram under traditional method incurred maximum expenditure on fertilizers (Rs. 1848), followed by seed and sowing (Rs. 1681), pesticides (Rs. 1195), and intercultural operations (Rs. 1037).

Table 3.9 further revealed that by adoption of sprinkler technology for gram, as per the expectation, the highest (Rs. 588) amount could be saved on labour cost of irrigation followed by intercultural operations (Rs. 316), electricity charges (Rs. 230), and fertilizers (Rs. 224). However, cost incurred on FYM, seed and sowing, and land preparation in case of gram cultivation under sprinkler technology found on higher side if compared to traditional method.

Thus, from above observations it could be concluded that drip/sprinkler technology substantially reduced the expenditure on cultivation of sugarcane, grapes, and gram in Latur district.

Similar to that of Latur district, attempt was also made to ascertain the cost of sugarcane and grapes cultivation under drip technology vis-à-vis traditional method in Osmanabad district. Results are provided in Table 3.10.

From the table it is observed that per acre average cost of sugarcane cultivation under drip technology reported to

Table 3.9

Cost of Cultivation (Rs/acre) for Study Crops under Sprinkler in Latur District

S.N.	Item	Sugarcane			Grapes		
		Drip	Traditional	Saving	Drip	Traditional	Saving
1	Land preparation	3077.68	3151.14	73.46	981.82	977.27	(4.55
		(14.63)	(12.20)	(2.38)	(9.83)	(8.58)	(-0.46)
2	Seed and sowing	4631.73	4943.36	311.63	1881.36	1681.33	(200.03
		(22.02)	(19.13)	(6.73)	(18.85)	(14.76)	(-10.63)
3	Fertilizer	5124.27	5812.21	687.94	1624.64	1848.54	223.9
		(24.37)	(22.50)	(13.42)	(16.28)	(16.22)	(13.78
4	FYM	3362.51	3421.43	58.92	1136.77	927.81	(208.96
		(15.98)	(13.24)	(1.75)	(11.39)	(8.14)	(-18.38)
5	Pesticide	138.33	271.68	133.35	995.46	1195.12	199.66
		(0.66)	(1.05)	(96.40)	(9.97)	(10.49)	(20.08)
6	Intercultural operations	1664.92	2337.54	672.62	721.48	1037.17	315.69
		(7.92)	(9.05)	(40.40)	(7.23)	(9.10)	(43.75)
7	Irrigation	752.47	3025.26	2272.79	375.35	963.2	587.85
	a) labour	(3.58)	(11.71)	(302.04)	(3.76)	(8.46)	(156.61)
	b) Electricity	1812.83	2037.67	224.84	647.27	877.56	230.29
	charges	(8.62)	(7.89)	(12.40)	(6.48)	(7.70)	(35.58)
8	Harvesting	-	-	-	818.44	976.31	157.87
					(8.20)	(8.57)	(19.29)

9	Transportation & mktg.	-	-	-	562.73 (5.64)	603.87 (5.30)	41.14 (7.31)
10	Others	466.08 (2.22)	833.76 (3.23)	367.68 (78.88)	236.66 (2.37)	305.13 (2.68)	68.47 (28.93)
	Total	21030.8 (100.00)	25834.1 (100.00)	4803.23 (22.84)	9981.98 (100.00)	11393.3 (100.00)	1411.33 (14.14)

Figures in brackets indicate percentage to total and that for under 'saving' column indicates percentage of corresponding saving.

Source : Field study.

be Rs. 18685 compared to Rs. 23032 under traditional method. Hence, about Rs. 4346 (23%) were saved per acre by adoption of drip technology. However, across operations, percentage of cost incurred on sugarcane cultivation under drip technology was reported highest (22%) for seed and sowing followed by fertilizers (21%), land preparation (20%), and FYM (12%). Compared to this sugarcane under traditional method required maximum expenditure on fertilizers (22%), seed and sowing (18%), land preparation (16%), and labour cost of irrigation (11%).

Further, individual item-wise drip technology over traditional method helped to save on labour cost of irrigation (Rs. 1538), fertilizers (Rs. 1107), intercultural operations (Rs. 653), and electricity charges (Rs. 631) on per acre basis for sugarcane cultivation.

Table 3.10 further revealed that per acre average cost of grapes cultivation under drip technology was worked out to Rs. 98463 in Osmanabad district, while that for under traditional method it was Rs. 125792. As regarding item-wise percentage contribution to the total cost of grapes cultivation under drip technology, pesticides contributed highest (24%) share followed by fertilizers (20%), intercultural operations (10%), and transportation and marketing (9%). While that for traditional method major items of total cost were found similar in order to that of drip technology but with different percentages.

As regarding saving by adoption of drip technology for grapes, sample farmers could saved about Rs. 27329 (28%) per acre over traditional method. However, item-wise savings was found highest (Rs. 10359) for pesticides followed by intercultural operations (Rs. 5959), labour cost of irrigation (Rs. 4935), fertilizers (Rs. 4312), and charges of electricity (Rs. 1298). Contrary to this, cost incurred on grapes cultivation under drip technology was found on higher side in case of transportation and marketing (Rs. 612), harvesting (Rs. 424), and seed and sowing (Rs. 229).

Thus, from above observations it could be inferred that expenditure incurred under traditional method of irrigation is more than drip irrigation. Further, unlike surface method of irrigation, drip does not encourage any growth of weed and hence helps in reduction of costs to be incurred on intercultural operations.

Table 3.11 depicts cost of sugarcane and gram cultivations under sprinkler technology vis-à-vis traditional method in Osmanabad district. As observed from the table per acre average cost of sugarcane cultivation under sprinkler technology worked out to be Rs. 20307 compared to Rs. 24637 as under traditional method. Thus, about Rs. 4330 (21%)/acre could be saved in sugarcane cultivation because of adoption of sprinkler technology in Osmanabad district. Across various items of cost of sugarcane cultivation under sprinkler technology fertilizers contributed highest (25%) share to the total cost followed by seed and sowing (22%), land preparation (15%), and FYM (12%). As regarding traditional method, major item to the total cost was fertilizers (22%) followed by seed and sowing (18%), FYM (13%), land preparation and labour cost of irrigation (12% each).

Further, except cost incurred on land preparation, and seed and sowing, sprinkler technology over traditional method for sugarcane reduced cost of all items under consideration. However, item-wise savings analysis revealed the maximum (Rs. 2061) savings in labour cost of irrigation followed by intercultural operations (Rs. 885), FYM (Rs. 626), and fertilizers (Rs. 397).

Average cost of gram cultivation under sprinkler technology in Osmanabad district worked out to be Rs. 8589 compared to Rs. 10558 under traditional method and thus reduced the cost by Rs. 1969/acre. However, item-wise maximum cost in gram cultivation under sprinkler technology was incurred on fertilizers, and seed and sowing (20% each) followed by FYM (12%), and land preparation (10%). While that for traditional method it was fertilizers, and seed and

Table 3.10
Cost of Cultivation (Rs/acre) for Study Crops under Drip in Osmanabad District

S.N.	Item	Sugarcane			Grapes		
		Drip	Traditional	Saving	Drip	Traditional	Saving
1	Land preparation	3751.9	3672.24	(79.66	5177.78	5804.11	626.33
		(20.08)	(15.94)	(-2.12)	(5.26)	(4.61)	(12.10)
2	Seed and sowing	4159.52	4088.1	(71.42	8214.44	7985.76	(228.68
		(22.26)	(17.75)	(-1.72)	(8.34)	(6.35)	(-2.78)
3	Fertilizer	3897.86	5004.76	1106.9	19876.7	24188.9	4312.22
		(20.86)	(21.73)	(28.40)	(20.19)	(19.23)	(21.69)
4	FYM	2289.29	2436.67	147.38	6188.89	7112.42	923.53
		(12.25)	(10.58)	(6.44)	(6.28)	(5.66)	(14.92)
5	Pesticide	142.86	157.14	14.28	23794.5	34153.1	10358.7
		(0.76)	(0.68)	(10.00)	(24.17)	(27.15)	(43.53)
6	Intercultural	1131.43	1784.29	652.86	10210.4	16168.9	5958.52
	operations	(6.06)	(7.75)	(57.70)	(10.37)	(12.85)	(58.36)
7	Irrigation	1072.38	2610.48	1358.1	2268.89	7204.34	4935.45
	a) labour	(5.74)	(11.34)	(143.43)	(2.30)	(5.73)	(217.53)
	b) Electricity	1686.43	2317.14	630.71	3740.18	5038.17	1297.99
	charges	(9.03)	(10.06)	(37.40)	(3.80)	(4.01)	(34.70)
8	Harvesting	-	-	-	8604.44	8180.08	(424.36
					(8.74)	(6.50)	(4.93)

9	Transportation & mktg.	-	-	-	9330.53	8718.91	(611.62
					(9.48)	(6.93)	(6.55)
10	Others	553.81	960.95	407.14	1056.67	1237.75	181.08
		(2.96)	(4.17)	(73.52)	(1.07)	(0.98)	(17.14)
	Total	18685.5	23031.8	4346.29	98463.3	125792	27329.1
		(100.00)	(100.00)	(23.26)	(100.00)	(100.00)	(27.75)

Figures in brackets indicate percentage to total and that for under 'saving' column indicates percentage of corresponding saving.
Source : Field study.

Table 3.11

Cost of Cultivation (Rs/acre) for Study Crops under Sprinkler in Osmanabad District

S.N.	Item	Sugarcane			Gram		
		Sprinkler	Traditional	Saving	Sprinkler	Traditional	Saving
1	Land preparation	3123.86	3047.75	(76.11	880.77	908.46	27.69
		(15.38)	(12.37)	(-2.44)	(10.25)	(8.60)	(3.14)
2	Seed and sowing	4550.04	4358.18	(191.86	1703.85	1823.08	119.23
		(22.41)	(17.69)	(-4.22)	(19.84)	(17.27)	(7.00)
3	Fertilizer	5030.43	5427.14	396.71	1726.15	1840.1	113.95
		(24.77)	(22.03)	(7.88)	(20.10)	(17.43)	(6.60)
4	FYM	2453.57	3079.29	625.72	1034.62	828.92	(205.7
		(12.08)	(12.50)	(25.50)	(12.05)	(7.85)	((19.88)
5	Pesticide	214.29	277.25	62.96	580.33	1076.02	495.69
		(1.06)	(1.12)	(29.38)	(6.76)	(10.19)	(85.41)
6	Intercultural operations	1332.16	2217.61	885.45	700.38	995.38	295
		(6.56)	(9.00)	(66.47)	(8.15)	(9.43)	(42.12)
7	Irrigation	882.06	2942.93	2060.87	245.42	893.85	648.43
	a) labour	(4.34)	(11.95)	(233.64)	(2.86)	(8.47)	(264.21)
	b) Electricity charges	2013.37	2192.37	179	304.23	653.51	349.28
		(9.92)	(8.90)	(8.89)	(3.54)	(6.19)	(114.81)
8	Harvesting	-	-	-	753.46	810.22	56.76
					(8.77)	(7.67)	(7.53)

9	Transportation & mktg.	-	-	-	495.77 (5.77)	509.43 (4.82)	13.66 (2.75)
10	Others	707.14 (3.48)	1094.29 (4.44)	387.15 (54.75)	164.23 (1.91)	219.18 (2.08)	54.95 (33.46)
	Total	20306.9 (100.00)	24636.8 (100.00)	4329.89 (21.32)	8589.21 (100.00)	10558.2 (100.00)	1968.94 (22.92)

Figures in brackets indicate percentage to total and that for under 'saving' column indicates percentage of corresponding saving.

Source : Field study.

sowing (17% each) followed by pesticides (10%), and intercultural operations (9%).

However, item-wise savings in gram cultivation by adoption of sprinkler technology revealed the maximum saving in labour cost of irrigation (Rs. 648) followed by pesticides (Rs. 496), electricity charges (Rs. 349), and intercultural operations (Rs. 295).

Thus, foregoing analysis revealed that compared to traditional method, drip/sprinkler technology substantially reduced the expenditure on cultivation of sugarcane, grapes, and gram in both the districts. However, except grapes and gram under sprinkler technology in Osmanabad district, amount of savings in all study crops under drip/sprinkler technology in Latur district was found on higher side than that of Osmanabad district. Further, unlike surface method of irrigation, drip does not encourage any growth of weed and hence helps in reduction of costs to be incurred on intercultural operations. Optimum use of costly chemical fertilizers through fertigation (under drip) and avoiding wastage (under both technologies) further helped farmers to save the money compared to the practices followed under traditional method. Great amount of labour and associated costs of irrigation could be saved by avoiding operations like control of water supply, changing course of water, governing leakages and seepages which are necessary in traditional method of irrigation. At the backdrop of heavy load shedding, savings in charges of electricity could be realized because of ability of drip/sprinkler technology to irrigate larger area in short period of time of power supply besides saving the valuable crops.

Maximum savings on labour cost of irrigation and intercultural operations across study crops under both the technologies indicates the tendency of farmers towards excessive use of costly inputs in the anticipation of higher yield. Hence, awareness and training for optimum utilization of inputs is in order.

3.9 Productivity

An attempt has been made to understand the yield difference of study crops between drip/sprinkler technology and traditional method of irrigation. Obtained results are provided in Table 3.12.

From the table it could be observed that the productivity is significantly higher for the sample farmers growing study crops under drip/sprinkler technology compared to traditional method of both the districts. Further, across districts and study crops productivity of all crops under both the technologies in Latur district was found on higher side compared to that of Osmanabad district. However, percentage increase in productivity over traditional method was reported higher in Osmanabad district for all study crops under the respective technology, except sugarcane under drip technology. This was mainly because of scarcity of water performance of water saving technologies (drip/sprinkler) was found much better and hence indicates further scope and need for these technologies in the study districts.

Among the crops under consideration sugarcane is being cultivated under both the technologies in the study districts. Analysis revealed that among both the districts productivity of sugarcane under drip technology was found higher than that of sprinkler technology. This was because of unlike surface method of irrigation drip does not encourage any growth of weed which ultimately helped to increase the yield of crops. Weeds, besides increasing labour cost on weeding, consume considerable amount of yield increasing inputs and reduce the yield of crop in traditional method of irrigation.

Thus, from the above observations it could be maintained that expenditure incurred under traditional method on different yield increasing inputs for crops under consideration, is more than that of under drip/sprinkler technology. However, this does not translated into increase in productivity of the respective study crops. Hence, it could be concluded that reported increase in productivity of crops under

Table 3.12

Per Acre Productivity (qtl/acre) of Study Crops

S.N.	Crop/unit	Latur			Osmanabad		
		Drip	Traditional	% Increase	Drip	Traditional	% Increase
1	Sugarcane	45.43	32.88	38.17	41.29	30.32	36.18
2	Grapes	129.13	103.58	24.67	107.78	86.11	25.16
		Sprinkler	Traditional	% increase	Sprinkler	Traditional	% increase
1	Sugarcane	39.25	33.67	16.57	37.53	29.41	27.61
2	Gram	8.18	6.67	22.64	7.95	6.13	29.7

Source : Field study.

consideration in the study districts is because of drip/sprinkler technology.

3.10 Comparative Economics

In order to judge the economic profitability of different crops under consideration per acre costs and returns were worked out and compared across the study districts. Further, to assess economic viability of crops, Income:Expenditure (I:E) ratios, i.e., returns per rupee invested were also worked out. The findings of the same for drip and sprinkler technology over traditional method are presented in Table 3.13 and 3.14 respectively.

Table 3.13 revealed that at overall level per acre average total cost and total income of sugarcane under drip technology were in the order of Rs. 19057 and Rs. 41059 respectively while for traditional method it were Rs. 24968 and Rs. 29921 respectively. This indicates higher expenditure and lower income realization in sugarcane cultivation under traditional method compared to drip technology. Further, per acre average net income realized by sugarcane under drip found significantly higher (Rs. 22002) compared to traditional method (Rs. 4953). The resultant I:E ratio for sugarcane under drip reported to be 2.15 compared to 1.20 under traditional method indicated that the sample farmers earned additional income to the tune of 1.15 over per rupee invested in sugarcane under drip technology as against Rs. 0.20 only in traditional method.

Further, across study districts total cost incurred and income realized in case of sugarcane under drip in Latur district were found on higher side than that of in Osmanabad district. Per acre net income of sugarcane under drip in Latur district worked out to be Rs. 24054 compared to Rs. 19950 in Osmanabad district. Resultant I:E ratios for Latur and Osmanabad districts for sugarcane under drip worked out to be 2.24 and 2.07 respectively over 1.17 and 1.23 respectively under traditional method indicating significant additional income generation by adoption of drip technology.

Table 3.13
Comparative Economics (Rs/acre) for Study Crops under Drip

S.N.	District	Item	Sugarcane		Grapes	
			Drip	Traditional	Drip	Traditional
1	Latur	Total cost	19428.57	26904.75	119374.77	144199.92
		Total income	43482.87	31470.76	254896.16	185225.90
		Net income	24054.30	4566.01	135521.39	41025.98
		I:E ratio	2.24	1.17	2.13	1.28
2	Osmanabad	Total cost	18685.48	23031.77	98463.31	125792.45
		Total income	38635.46	28370.73	222745.70	177960.95
		Net income	19949.98	5338.96	124282.39	52168.50
		I:E ratio	2.07	1.23	2.26	1.14
3	Average	Total cost	19057.02	24968.26	108919.04	134996.18
		Total income	41059.16	29920.74	238820.93	181593.42
		Net income	22002.14	4952.48	129901.89	46597.24
		I:E ratio	2.15	1.20	2.19	1.34

Source : Field study.

Table 3.14
Comparative Economics (Rs/acre) for Study Crops under Sprinkler

S.N.	District	Item	Sugarcane		Grapes	
			Sprinkler	Traditional	Sprinkler	Traditional
1	Latur	Total cost	21030.82	25834.05	9981.98	11393.31
		Total income	34835.16	29882.80	16657.42	12894.71
		Net income	13804.34	4048.75	6675.44	1501.40
		I:E ratio	1.66	1.16	1.67	1.13
2	Osmanabad	Total cost	20306.92	24636.81	8589.21	10558.15
		Total income	34510.67	27015.14	15655.38	12324.61
		Net income	14203.75	2378.33	7066.17	1766.46
		I:E ratio	1.70	1.10	1.82	1.17
3	Average	Total cost	20668.87	25235.43	9285.60	10975.73
		Total income	34672.91	28448.97	16156.40	12609.66
		Net income	14004.04	3213.54	6870.80	1633.93
		I:E ratio	1.68	1.13	1.74	1.15

Source : Field study.

Thus, the positive returns on investments and more than unity I:E ratios indicated that sugarcane under both the methods (drip/sprinkler) was an economically viable crop for the sample farmers. However, the level of profitability for sugarcane under drip technology was much higher if compared with traditional method.

Similar to the trends observed for sugarcane in Latur district, grapes also exhibited higher expenditure and lower income realization under traditional method over drip technology at overall level. However, compared to sugarcane under drip the amount of net income realization per acre by grapes under drip was found significantly higher (Rs. 129902) than traditional method (Rs. 46597). Subsequent I:E ratios for grapes under drip as well as traditional method were worked out to be 2.19 and 1.34 respectively indicating much higher returns on each rupee invested in grapes under drip technology.

Across districts, grapes under drip technology in Latur reported higher (Rs. 135521) net income per acre than that of Rs. 124282 in Osmanabad district. However, resultant I:E ratio in Osmanabad district was found on higher side (2.16) than Latur district (2.13). This was because per acre cost incurred on grape cultivation under drip in Osmanabad district was found comparatively less (Rs. 98463) than that of Latur district (Rs. 119375).

From above observations it could be concluded that grape was an economically viable crop under drip as well as traditional method of irrigation for sample farmers of study districts, but comparatively more profitable under drip technology.

It could be observed from Table 3.14 that sugarcane under sprinkler technology incurred less cost (Rs. 20669) compared to traditional method (Rs. 25235) on per acre basis. Further, owing to better productivity, per acre total income, net income, and resultant I:E ratio obtained for sugarcane under sprinkler technology were found significantly higher (Rs. 34673, Rs.

14004, and 1.68 respectively) than that of under traditional method (Rs. 28449, Rs. 3214, and 1.13 respectively). Similar trend was observed across the study districts for sugarcane but with different values for parameters under consideration. Across districts per acre net income realization and I:E ratio obtained for sugarcane under sprinkler technology in Osmanabad district were found on higher side (Rs. 14204 and 1.70 respectively) compared to Latur district (Rs. 13804 and 1.66 respectively). This indicates comparatively better utilization of scare water in Osmanabad district through water saving sprinkler technology.

Thus, from the obtained positive returns and better I:E ratios, one could infer that sugarcane under sprinkler as well as under traditional method was an economically viable crop among study districts. However, the amount of profitability under sprinkler over traditional method was found significantly higher. Further, across water saving technologies (drip and sprinkler) per acre net income realization in case of sugarcane was found significantly higher for drip technology compared to sprinkler technology. This was mainly because of drip technology's advantages over sprinkler technology like checking growth of weed, allowing fertigation, and irrigating larger area within short period of time.

Table 3.14 further revealed that gram under traditional method incurred higher cost (Rs. 10976) and lower net income (Rs. 1634) compared to that of Rs. 9286 and Rs. 6871 respectively under sprinkler technology at overall level. Resultant I:E ratio for gram under sprinkler technology was found on higher side (1.74) compared to traditional method (1.15) indicating much better returns on each rupee invested in gram under sprinkler technology. Across study districts, Osmanabad district reported lower cost (Rs. 8589) and higher (Rs. 7066) net income for gram under sprinkler technology than that for Rs. 9982 and Rs. 6675 respectively in Latur district. Accordingly, resultant I:E ratio for gram under sprinkler technology was found on higher side (1.82) in Osmanabad district compared to that of Latur district's (1.67). Compared to this I:E ratios obtained for gram under traditional method were reported much lower indicating significant impact of sprinkler technology on cost savings.

From above observations, it could be summed-up that the crops under consideration incurred more cost on per acre basis under traditional method of irrigation as compared to drip/sprinkler technology. This was because of several advantages of drip/sprinkler like efficient use of water and critical inputs, lesser weed problems and associated costs, and ability to irrigate larger area within short period of time compared to traditional method of irrigation. In effect, average production and hence resultant net income obtained by crops grown under water saving technologies was found to be on higher side than traditional method. The positive profitability measures and more than one I:E ratios obtained in all crops under drip/sprinkler technology as well as traditional method indicates that farming of these crops in study districts is economically profitable and viable. However, depending on nature of crop (grapes over sugarcane and sugarcane over gram), and method of irrigation (drip and sprinkler over traditional method, and drip over sprinkler) the level of profitability was found significantly higher.

3.11 Uncertainty in Production

Uncertainty refers to future events wherein the parameters of profitability distribution cannot be determined empirically or quantitatively. It is very difficult to measure the uncertainty with any acceptable degree of accuracy. However, an attempt has been made to estimate the yield and price uncertainty ratios in study crops on before and after adoption of technology basis; as an empirical measure of degree of uncertainty. The study adopted methodology followed by Chandel, *et. al.* (1997), Dixit, *et. al.* (1999), and Dileep, *et.al.* (2002).

3.11.1 Yield Uncertainty Ratio

The yield uncertainty ratios of study crops under drip and sprinkler technology against traditional method were worked out and the results are provided in Table 3.15 and Table 3.16 respectively.

It is evident from Table 3.15 that at overall level yield uncertainty was generally lower for sugarcane (0.28) and grapes (0.38) under drip technology as compared to before adoption of this technology. Across study crops, yield uncertainty prior to adoption of drip technology was reported higher for grapes in Latur (0.72) and Osmanabad (0.66) district compared to sugarcane (0.54 and 0.57 respectively) in both the districts. Scarcity of water, limitations on use of water owing to load shedding, weed infestation, and wastage of scarce water under traditional method of irrigation leads to higher yield uncertainties among study crops. As against this, owing to adoption of drip technology above mentioned disadvantages reduces significantly and helped to achieve certain amount of stability in productivity. Accordingly, yield uncertainty across study crops under drip worked out to be lesser for sugarcane in Latur (0.25) and Osmanabad (0.32) district compared to grapes (0.42 and 0.34 respectively) among both the districts.

Further, yield uncertainties in study crops under sprinkler technology were found on higher side compared to that of under drip technology (Table 3.16). Yield uncertainty at overall level for gram was found to be high during before and after adoption of technology and worked out to be 0.78 and 0.47 respectively. Compared to this the same for sugarcane worked out to be 0.56 and 0.32 respectively. Across districts similar trends were reported for both the districts but with different values. Before adoption of sprinkler technology, highest yield uncertainty was reported for gram (0.84) in Osmanabad district and that for sugarcane (0.58) in Latur district. This was because of above mentioned disadvantages of traditional method of

Table 3.15
Minimization of Yield Uncertainty under Drip

S.	Crop	Particular	Latur		Osmanabad		Average	
			Before	After	Before	After	Before	After
1	Sugarcane (quintal/acre)	Highest yield obtained	33.12	49.43	35.10	47.90	34.11	48.66
		Most probable yield	25.57	43.29	29.33	41.10	27.45	42.19
		Lowest yield obtained	19.29	38.71	18.43	34.88	18.86	36.79
		Yield uncertainty	0.54	0.25	0.57	0.32	0.55	0.28
2	Grapes (quintal/acre)	Highest yield obtained	94.78	163.04	88.24	136.67	91.51	149.85
		Most probable yield	70.22	127.83	64.81	115.56	67.51	121.69
		Lowest yield obtained	43.91	109.67	45.72	97.22	44.81	103.44
		Yield uncertainty	0.72	0.42	0.66	0.34	0.69	0.38

Source : Field study.

Table 3.16

Minimization of Yield Uncertainty under Sprinkler

SN	Crop	Particular	Latur		Osmanabad		Average	
			Before	After	Before	After	Before	After
1	Sugarcane (quintal/acre)	Highest yield obtained	35.13	41.37	36.44	44.53	35.78	42.95
		Most probable yield	24.15	34.41	30.53	39.29	27.34	36.85
		Lowest yield obtained	21.04	29.85	20.14	32.57	20.59	31.21
		Yield uncertainty	0.58	0.33	0.53	0.30	0.56	0.32
2	Gram (quintal/acre)	Highest yield obtained	7.12	9.35	6.46	8.84	6.80	9.10
		Most probable yield	5.21	7.62	4.52	7.17	4.86	7.40
		Lowest yield obtained	3.32	5.91	2.67	5.37	3.00	5.64
		Yield uncertainty	0.73	0.45	0.84	0.48	0.78	0.47

Source : Field study.

irrigation. Further, by adoption of sprinkler technology sample farmers realized lesser amount of yield uncertainty in sugarcane (0.30 in Osmanabad and 0.33 in Latur district), and gram (0.45 in Latur and 0.48 in Osmanabad district). Thus, by adoption of sprinkler technology sample farmers could irrigate more area within short period of time as well as could be able to provide protective irrigations during critical growth stages of study crops and hence able to stabilize the production of study crops.

From above observations it could be concluded that yield uncertainty of crops under consideration in study districts were minimized significantly by virtue of increased production through adoption of water saving drip/sprinkler technology as compared to traditional method of irrigation. Further, across technology, comparatively yield uncertainty in study crops under drip technology reported minimum than that of under sprinkler technology in the study area.

3.11.2 *Price Uncertainty Ratio*

The price uncertainty ratios of study crops under drip and sprinkler technologies in comparison with traditional method of irrigation were calculated and the results obtained are presented in Table 3.17 and Table 3.18 respectively.

Price offered to agricultural produce is subjected to wide fluctuations owing to nature of crop, perishability, prevailing market conditions, etc. Improvement in quality is to be considered as one of the main advantage of drip/sprinkler technology. Ultimately this helps farmers to fetch better and assured price for their produce and hence help to cope up with wide price uncertainty to some extent.

It could be seen from Table 3.17 that the highest price uncertainty ratio (0.57) was observed in grapes before adoption of drip technology followed by sugarcane (0.35) at overall level. Compared to this after adoption of drip the lowest price uncertainty ratio (0.17) was observed in sugarcane followed by grapes (0.42) at overall level. Crops under

Table 3.17
Minimization of Price Uncertainty under Drip

S.N.	Crop	Particular	Latur		Osmanabad		Average	
			Before	After	Before	After	Before	After
1	Sugarcane (Rs./tonne)	Highest price obtained	707.14	1064.29	730.95	1010.72	719.04	1037.50
		Most probable price	592.86	933.45	600.81	930.95	596.83	932.20
		Lowest price obtained	514.29	892.86	506.19	869.05	510.24	880.95
		Price uncertainty	0.33	0.18	0.37	0.15	0.35	0.17
2	Grapes (Rs./quintal)	Highest price obtained	1404.35	2395.65	1311.12	2550.18	1357.73	2472.91
		Most probable price	1034.78	1923.11	961.02	1887.67	997.90	1905.39
		Lowest price obtained	832.61	1626.08	745.14	1722.37	788.87	1674.22
		Price uncertainty	0.55	0.40	0.59	0.44	0.57	0.42

Source : Field study.

consideration across study districts exhibited similar trends but with different values. However, minimization of price uncertainty in sugarcane is reported much better than grapes. Besides political reasons, increased productivity of sugarcane by means of adoption of drip technology helped the sugar factories operating in the study area to utilize their plant capacity fully and hence to realize better income and better price to farmers. While for grapes, besides assured and increased yield levels, improvement in quality helped sample farmers to tap foreign markets and hence better price to their produce.

Further, before adoption of sprinkler technology price uncertainty ratios in gram and sugarcane were worked out to be 0.41 and 0.35 respectively which further minimized substantially to the tune of 0.34 and 0.20 respectively at overall level after adoption of the technology (Table 3.18). Across districts and crops under consideration, price uncertainty ratio before adoption of sprinkler technology was reported highest (0.43) for gram in Osmanabad district and for sugarcane (0.36) in Latur district. After adoption of sprinkler technology sample farmers minimized price uncertainty in study crops significantly. Crop-wise lowest price uncertainty ratio was reported for gram (0.30) in Latur district and that for sugarcane (0.33) in Osmanabad district. Further, across technology adopted price uncertainty ratio in sugarcane under sprinkler technology was found slightly more than that of drip technology. Reasons behind minimized price uncertainty of sugarcane under sprinkler technology are similar to that of drip technology. While for gram it was because of increased yield of the crop farmers could store part of production and sold them in market after some time at better prices by means of avoiding glut and very low prices occurred immediate after harvest of the produce.

Thus, from above observations it could be inferred that price uncertainty in study crops could be minimized significantly by means of assured and increased production

Table 3.18
Minimization of Price Uncertainty under Sprinkler

S.N.	Crop	Particular	Latur		Osmanabad		Average	
			Before	After	Before	After	Before	After
1	Sugarcane (Rs./ tonne)	Highest price obtained	783.25	960.23	757.14	988.11	770.19	974.17
		Most probable price	612.18	848.51	635.71	905.75	623.94	877.13
		Lowest price obtained	565.61	767.44	542.86	821.43	554.23	794.43
		Price uncertainty	0.36	0.22	0.33	0.18	0.35	0.20
2	Gram (Rs./ quintal)	Highest price obtained	1972.51	2081.82	1892.31	2130.13	1932.41	2105.97
		Most probable price	1622.03	1724.11	1652.38	1808.13	1637.20	1766.12
		Lowest price obtained	1354.78	1563.46	1180.77	1450.24	1267.77	1506.85
		Price uncertainty	0.38	0.30	0.43	0.38	0.41	0.34

Source : Field study.

through adoption of drip/sprinkler technology. However, across technology, minimization of price uncertainty in study crops under drip technology found slightly better than that of under sprinkler technology in the study area.

3.12 Capital and Production Cost

For rapid diffusion of capital intensive drip/sprinkler technology among farmers government provides 50% of the capital cost as subsidy to the willing farmers. High cost of such sets, especially that of drip, increased the production cost and hence subsidy plays important role in the amount of profit earned. In a given situation an attempt has been made to understand the per acre level of profit earned by study crops cultivated under drip and sprinkler technology. Obtained results are provided in Table 3.19.

It could be observed from the table that across districts per acre capital cost of drip set ranged between Rs. 51533 for grapes in Osmanabad district to Rs. 44075 for sugarcane in Latur district indicating higher capital cost for grapes cultivators. While that for sprinkler set it varied between Rs. 20846 for sugarcane in Osmanabad district to Rs. 18862 for gram in Latur district. Further, production costs as well as gross value of production of crops under consideration cultivated under drip and sprinkler in Latur district reported to be on higher side than that of in Osmanabad district. Regarding the profit without subsidy, except grapes under drip, all study crops under both the technologies reported negative returns in the study districts indicates the necessity of subsidy provision for economical and effective adoption of the technologies. Being a highly remunerative crop, grapes cultivators comfortably afford the capital cost of drip set. Hence, the profit with subsidy for grapes under drip reported highest among both the study districts across crops under consideration. Further, the amount of profit with subsidy for study crops under drip technology were found on higher side in Latur district and that for crops under sprinkler technology in Osmanabad district.

Table 3.19
Capital and Production Cost (Rs.) in Study Districts

S.N.	Particular	Drip		Sprinkler	
		Sugarcane	Grapes	Sugarcane	Gram
	Latur				
1	Capital cost of set	44075.30	45603.14	19125.26	18861.85
2	Production cost	19428.57	119374.77	21030.82	9981.98
3	Gross value of production	43482.87	254896.16	34835.16	16657.42
4	Profit without subsidy	- 20021.00	89918.25	- 5320.92	- 12186.41
5	Profit with subsidy	24054.30	135521.39	13804.34	6675.44
	Osmanabad				
1	Capital cost of set	49461.67	51533.21	20846.11	19135.43
2	Production cost	18685.48	98463.31	20306.92	8589.21
3	Gross value of production	38635.46	222745.70	34510.67	15655.38
4	Profit without subsidy	- 29511.69	72749.18	- 6642.36	- 12069.26
5	Profit with subsidy	19949.98	124282.39	14203.75	7066.17

Source : Field study.

Thus, from above observations it could be concluded that per acre capital cost of drip set compared to sprinkler set is quite high and hence substantially increased the production cost and significantly reduced the profit margin. Further, subsidy administration is necessary for partial recovery of increased production cost to obtain better profit from crops grown under these technologies.

3.13 Summary

Performance of MIS at field level is analyzed in this chapter. Majority of adopters were educated and belonged to medium or large land holdings with irrigation facilities. Sugarcane under drip contributed highest share in Osmanabad while grapes in Latur. Sprinkler technology is found popular in Latur and drip in Osmanabad for cultivation of cash crops (sugarcane, grapes, vegetables, fruit crops, etc). Prolonged power cuts, less water requirement, subsidy, reduction in cost of cultivation, labour saving, and increase in yield were the factors influencing adoption of improved technology. Sample farmers mostly contacted dealers to solve their problems.

Due to ignorance majority of farmers from both the districts could not verify quality assurance marks. Negative correlation was reported between size of land holding and average investment made in drip/sprinkler. Sprinkler adopters invested comparatively more of own funds over bank loans than drip adopters. Problem of non-functioning of MI sets is major for drip adopters of Osmanabad.

Drip/sprinkler technology substantially reduced the expenditure on cultivation of sugarcane, grapes, and gram in both the districts. Productivity is found significantly higher for farmers growing crops under drip/sprinkler technology compared to traditional method. Contrarily, expenditure incurred under traditional method on different yield increasing inputs was found more than that under drip/sprinkler technology. It could be concluded that productivity increase was mainly due to drip/sprinkler technology. The positive profitability measures and more than one I:E ratios obtained in all crops under drip/sprinkler technology as well as traditional method indicate reasonable returns from farming. However, depending on nature of crop (grapes over sugarcane and sugarcane over gram), and method of irrigation (drip and sprinkler over traditional method, and drip over sprinkler) the level of profitability was found significantly higher.

Yield uncertainties of crops in study area were minimized significantly by virtue of increased productivity through adoption of water saving technology. Comparatively yield uncertainty under drip technology reported minimum than that under sprinkler technology. Highest price uncertainty ratio was observed in grapes followed by sugarcane before adoption of water saving technology. Per acre capital cost of drip set is more and hence substantially increased the cost of production. Subsidy administration is necessary for partial recovery of increased production cost to obtain profit from crops grown under these technologies.

4
Impact of Micro-irrigation on Input Use

Previous chapter dealt with how drip/sprinkler reduces cost of cultivation and increases productivity of crops. Besides this, these technologies help to save water and improve water use efficiency. While doing so it also reduces substantial amount of electricity required for irrigation by reducing working hours of irrigation pumpsets. In the light of limited studies on water saving and electricity saving at farm level data owing to micro-irrigation an attempt has been made to assess the same in the study districts. Methodology adopted for estimation of consumption of water and electricity is heavily based on Shah (1993), and Narayanamoorthy (2005).

4.1 Crop-wise Water Use Pattern

Water use pattern refers to number of irrigation used, hours required to irrigate, pumpset (HP), etc. Further, it varies with the source of irrigation and crops to be irrigated. Since the sample farmers mainly using groundwater and able to control water supply, water use pattern obviously may not be the same as that of flood method of irrigation. Hence attempt has been made to analyze crop-wise water use pattern in the study districts and results are provided in Table 4.1.

It could be observed from the table that the numbers of irrigations used per acre under drip/sprinkler technology for crops under consideration are higher than that of under traditional method of irrigation at overall level. For example, on an average in sugarcane and grapes under drip technology sample farmers irrigated nearly 23 times and 48 times respectively more than the traditional method. Likewise, in sugarcane and gram under sprinkler technology the corresponding figures are 17 times and 1 time respectively. Across technologies and study crops frequency of irrigation was found relatively higher for grapes and sugarcane under drip than sugarcane and gram under sprinkler technology. Further, district-wise analysis revealed that frequency of irrigations in study crops under drip as well as traditional method was found on higher side in Latur district than Osmanabad district, while that for sprinkler technology, except sugarcane in Latur district, the corresponding figures were found on higher side in Osmanabad district than Latur district. However, across districts individual crop-wise frequency of irrigation under drip technology over traditional method for grapes and sugarcane in Latur district reported higher (61 times and 29 times respectively) than Osmanabad district (35 times and 17 times respectively), while that for sugarcane under sprinkler in Latur and Osmanabad districts reported 25 times and 10 times more than traditional method of irrigation. The corresponding figures for gram crop were reported marginally higher over traditional method. In order to maintain the moisture level under acute water scarcity and ability to irrigate larger area in limited hours of electricity available, sample farmers having drip/sprinkler technology used water at required frequency. Therefore the actual numbers of irrigations used by them are relatively higher than traditional method of irrigation.

Table 4.1 further revealed that despite more number of

Table 4.1
Per Acre Crop-wise Water Use Pattern

S.N.	Crop	Particular	Latur		Osmanabad		Average	
			Drip	Traditional	Drip	Traditional	Drip	Traditional
1	Sugarcane	Number of irrigations	116.32	87.46	101.83	84.60	109.07	86.03
		Number of hours system used	4.33	8.49	5.19	8.67	4.76	8.58
		Pump set (HP)	5.71	6.25	5.55	5.90	5.63	6.07
2	Grapes	Number of irrigations	163.51	102.23	129.44	94.48	146.47	98.35
		Number of hours system used	4.73	8.58	4.56	9.12	4.64	8.85
		Pump set (HP)	4.83	6.12	6.11	5.83	5.47	5.97
	Crop	Particular	Sprinkler	Traditional	Sprinkler	Traditional	Sprinkler	Traditional
1	Sugarcane	Number of irrigations	98.66	73.66	85.57	76.27	92.11	74.96
		Number of hours system used	7.53	12.07	7.66	9.35	7.60	10.71
		Pump set (HP)	5.28	5.93	5.21	6.21	5.24	6.07
2	Gram	Number of irrigations	2.14	1.52	2.54	2.13	2.34	1.82
		Number of hours system used	6.45	9.62	5.15	8.77	5.80	9.19
		Pump set (HP)	4.27	4.95	5.05	4.67	4.66	4.81

Source : Field study.

irrigations used for study crops under drip/sprinkler technology, the time utilized in hours per irrigation is significantly less for drip technology over sprinkler as well as traditional method of irrigation. Since drip method supplies water only at the root zone of the crop, time required per irrigation is much less. Contrary to this, under traditional method of irrigation uneven land surface, open conveying channels, evaporation losses, etc., significantly increases time as well as quantity of water consumption. However, among sprinkler and traditional method of irrigation, sprinkler technology required significantly less hours to irrigate the study crops than traditional method. Thus, with limited water and time period, drip/ sprinkler technology helped the sample farmers to maintain moisture level and avoid water stress for crops under consideration.

4.2 Water Consumption

Water consumption per acre for any crop is determined by factors like horse power of the pumpset, water level of the well, capacity of pump, size of delivery pipes, condition of the water extraction machineries, distance between place of water source and field to be irrigated, quality of soil, crop, terrain condition, etc. These factors vary considerably across farmers. Present study measured the water consumption in terms of water horse power (HP) hours of irrigation. HP hours of water is computed by multiplying HP of the pumpset with hours of system used for crops under consideration in the study district (Narayanamoorthy, 2005). Results are given in Table 4.2.

Table 4.2 reveals that per acre consumption of water in terms of HP hours for drip technology was found significantly less than sprinkler and traditional method of irrigation. For instance, per acre water consumption in sugarcane and grapes under drip reported to be 2923 and 3718 HP hours respectively compared to 4481 and 5196 HP hours respectively under traditional method. Likewise, for sugarcane and gram under

Table 4.2
Per Acre Water Consumption (HP hour/acre)

S.N.	Crop	Latur		Osmanabad		Average	
		Drip	Traditional	Drip	Traditional	Drip	Traditional
1	Sugarcane	2875.93	4640.85	2933.16	4327.54	2922.94	4480.50
2	Grapes	3735.53	5368.06	3606.40	5023.46	3717.52	5196.27
	Crop	Sprinkler	Traditional	Sprinkler	Traditional	Sprinkler	Traditional
1	Sugarcane	3922.56	5272.22	3414.98	4428.50	3668.19	4873.13
2	Gram	58.94	72.38	66.06	87.24	63.24	80.45

Source : Field study.

sprinkler it was worked out to be 3668 and 63 HP hours respectively as compared to 4873 and 80 HP hours respectively in traditional method of irrigation. Study districts exhibited similar trends but with different figures. However, across districts and crops under consideration, grapes under drip as well as under traditional method consumed more water in Latur district compared to that of Osmanabad district. That for sugarcane under drip in Osmanabad district and sugarcane under traditional method in Latur district consumed more water on per acre basis to that of their counterparts. Further, per acre water consumption under sprinkler technology in sugarcane and gram reported significantly less than traditional method. However, across districts, per acre water consumption under sprinkler for sugarcane in Osmanabad district and for gram in Latur district reported less. Thus, from above observations it could be concluded that per acre water consumption under drip/sprinkler technology is much less than that of traditional method of irrigation.

4.3 Saving in Water Consumption

The requirement of water varies crop-wise and technology-wise depending upon the soil quality and other factors. Hence, to understand crop-wise and technology-wise actual percentage of saving of water consumption, HP hours, and additional area could be irrigate with that saved water and HP hours at farm level an attempt has been made to assess the same. Results are provided in Table 4.3.

It could be observed from the table that water savings in terms of percentage and HP hours were much higher for sugarcane under drip as compared to grapes. Further, across districts, per acre savings in water consumption under drip technology for study crops in Latur district were found on higher side than Osmanabad district. Accordingly, with the help of saved water under drip, sample farmers can bring 0.53 acres under sugarcane and 0.40 acres under grapes at overall level.

Table 4.3
Per Acre Saving in Water Consumption

S.N.	Particular	Latur		Osmanabad		Average	
		%	HP	%	HP	%	HP
Drip							
1	Sugarcane	61.37	1764.92	47.54	1394.38	53.29	1557.56
2	Grapes	43.70	1632.53	39.30	1417.06	39.78	1478.75
Additional area (acre) can be irrigated							
1	Sugarcane	0.61		0.47		0.53	
2	Grapes	0.44		0.39		0.40	
Sprinkler							
1	Sugarcane	34.41	1349.66	29.68	1013.52	32.85	1204.94
2	Gram	22.80	13.44	32.06	21.18	27.21	17.21
Additional area (acre) can be irrigated							
1	Sugarcane	0.34		0.30		0.33	
2	Gram	0.23		0.32		0.27	

Source : Field study.

Similar to that of drip technology, per acre water savings in percentage and HP hours were found significantly higher for sugarcane under sprinkler technology if compared to gram at overall level. Further, with the help of saved water sample farmers can bring 0.33 acres under sugarcane and 0.27 acres under gram at overall level. The result indicates that drip/sprinkler technology helps saving more water in water intensive crops like sugarcane and also in bringing more area under irrigation.

4.4 Per Quintal Water Consumption

To understand the importance of drip/sprinkler technology in increasing the efficiency of water use, per quintal water consumption in study crops were calculated. The arrived results are given in Table 4.4.

It could be observed from the table that sugarcane and grapes under drip technology consumed only 67.41 and 31.38 hours of water compared to 141.74 and 54.79 hours of water under traditional method to produce one quintal of yield at overall level. This indicates lower consumption of water under drip technology over traditional method of irrigation. Further, across districts and study crops, corresponding figures were reported much less in Latur district compared to Osmanabad district. Among study crops, sugarcane being water intensive crop required significantly higher amount of water than grapes.

Further, per quintal water consumption in HP hours for sugarcane and gram under sprinkler technology at overall level were found on lower side (95.55 and 7.85 hours respectively) than traditional method (154.51 and 12.57 hours respectively) indicating efficiency of sprinkler technology in water savings. Across districts, corresponding figures reported lower for sugarcane in Osmanabad district and that for gram in Latur district. Thus, the above observations clearly show that drip/sprinkler technology reduced the per acre consumption of water on per unit of crop yield basis.

Table 4.4

Water Consumption per Unit of Yield (HP hours/quintal)

SN	Crop	Latur		Osmanabad		Average	
		Drip	Traditional	Drip	Traditional	Drip	Traditional
1	Sugarcane	63.63	141.40	71.04	142.73	67.41	141.74
2	Grapes	28.93	51.82	33.46	58.34	31.38	54.79
	Crop	Sprinkler	Traditional	Sprinkler	Traditional	Sprinkler	Traditional
1	Sugarcane	99.94	156.58	91.00	150.58	95.55	154.51
2	Gram	7.20	10.85	8.31	14.23	7.85	12.57

Source : Field study.

4.5 Electricity Consumption

As indicated earlier that total working hours of pumpset in case of drip/sprinkler technology on per acre basis are less than traditional method of irrigation. Further, for estimating electricity it has been assumed that for every hour of operation 0.75 kwh of power is used per HP (Shah, 1993). Hence, to estimate per acre electricity consumption for study crops under respective method of irrigation, total HP hours are multiplied by 0.75/kwh/HP (Narayanamoorthy, 2005). The results are provided in Table 4.5.

Table 4.5 revealed that sample farmers using drip/sprinkler technology used very less amount of electricity for all crops under consideration compared to traditional method of irrigation owing to less number of operating hours of pumpsets. For instance, per acre electricity consumption in sugarcane and grapes under drip worked out to be 2192.20 and 2788.14 kwh respectively compared to 3360.37 and 3897.20 kwh respectively at overall level. Across districts, sugarcane in Latur district and grapes in Osmanabad district consumed less electricity on per acre basis compared to their counterparts.

That for sugarcane and gram under sprinkler technology per acre electricity consumption worked out to be 2751.14 and 47.43 kwh respectively compared to 3654.85 and 60.34 kwh respectively in traditional method of irrigation. Across districts sugarcane in Osmanabad district and gram in Latur district reported lower per acre consumption of electricity.

Thus, above observations revealed that owing to less operating hours of pumpsets, drip/sprinkler technology significantly reduces the consumption of electricity over traditional method of irrigation.

4.6 Saving in Electricity Consumption

Water requirement, number of irrigations, and hours of operating pumpset varies with crops, method of irrigation,

Table 4.5
Per Acre Electricity Consumption (KWH)

S.N.	Crop	Latur		Osmanabad		Average	
		Drip	Traditional	Drip	Traditional	Drip	Traditional
1	Sugarcane	2156.95	3480.64	2199.87	3245.65	2192.20	3360.37
2	Grapes	2801.65	4026.04	2704.80	3767.60	2788.14	3897.20
	Crop	**Sprinkler**	**Traditional**	**Sprinkler**	**Traditional**	**Sprinkler**	**Traditional**
1	Sugarcane	2941.92	3954.16	2561.23	3321.37	2751.14	3654.85
2	Gram	44.20	54.28	49.54	65.43	47.43	60.34

Source : Field study.

water and electricity availability, etc. Considering this an attempt has been made to estimate crop-wise and technology-wise actual savings of electricity in study area. The obtained results are provided in Table 4.6.

Table 4.6 shows that at overall level per acre savings in electricity consumption for sugarcane and grapes under drip technology worked out to be 1168.17 and 1109.06 kwh respectively over traditional method of irrigations. Compared to this the corresponding figures for sugarcane and gram under sprinkler technology were reported to be 903.70 and 12.91 kwh respectively. This indicates savings in electricity consumption in drip technology is much higher than sprinkler technology. Further, among crops under consideration, amount of electricity saving on per acre basis for sugarcane

Table 4.6
Per Acre Estimates of Electricity (KWH) Saved

SN	Crop	Latur	Osmanabad	Average
Drip				
1	Sugarcane	1323.69	1045.78	1168.17
2	Grapes	1224.40	1062.80	1109.06
Sprinkler				
1	Sugarcane	1012.24	760.14	903.70
2	Gram	10.08	15.88	12.91

Source : Field study.

under drip is found much more than remaining crops under respective method of irrigation. Being water intensive crop, requirement of water for sugarcane is much higher than other study crops. However, owing to less hours of pumpset operation under drip technology, the amount of electricity saved was reported significantly higher than others.

4.7 Per Quintal Electricity Consumption

In order to understand efficiency of electricity consumption, energy used to produce one quintal of yield is computed by dividing per acre energy consumption by yield and the results are presented in Table 4.7.

Table 4.7 shows that per quintal consumption of energy for study crops is quite low for drip/sprinkler technology compared to traditional method of irrigation. For instance, at overall level sugarcane and grapes under drip technology spend about 50.56 and 23.54 kwh respectively to produce one quintal of yield whereas the same was found much higher for traditional method and worked out to be 106.31 and 41.10 kwh respectively. That for sugarcane and gram under sprinkler technology worked out to be 71.66 and 5.88 kwh respectively compared to 115.88 and 9.43 kwh respectively under traditional method.

Further, across districts per acre electricity consumption in sugarcane and grapes under drip technology reported on lower side in Latur district than Osmanabad district. However, for sprinkler technology, sugarcane in Osmanabad district and gram in Latur district registered lower consumption of electricity on per acre basis than their counterparts.

From above observations it could be concluded that electricity consumption to produce one quintal of yield is significantly less in drip/sprinkler technology as compared to traditional method of irrigation.

4.8 Summary

Impact of micro-irrigation on water and electricity consumption was studied in this chapter. The number of irrigations provided under drip/sprinkler technology is higher than traditional method of irrigation. Frequency of irrigation was found relatively higher for grapes and sugarcane under drip than sugarcane and gram under sprinkler technology. With limited water and time period,

Table 4.7
Electricity Consumption (KWH) per Unit of Yield

S.N.	Crop	Latur		Osmanabad		Average	
		Drip	Traditional	Drip	Traditional	Drip	Traditional
1	Sugarcane	47.48	105.86	53.28	107.05	50.56	106.31
2	Grapes	21.70	38.87	25.10	43.75	23.54	41.10
	Crop	Sprinkler	Traditional	Sprinkler	Traditional	Sprinkler	Traditional
1	Sugarcane	74.95	117.44	68.24	112.93	71.66	115.88
2	Gram	5.40	8.14	6.23	10.67	5.88	9.43

Source : Field study.

drip/sprinkler technology helped farmers to maintain moisture level and avoid water stress for crops under consideration. Further, per acre consumption of water in terms of HP hours for drip technology was found significantly less than sprinkler and traditional method. Drip/sprinkler technology helped in saving water for sugarcane, and thus bringing more area under irrigation. Drip/sprinkler technology reduced water consumption per unit of yield (quintal).

Drip/sprinkler technology significantly reduced consumption of electricity over traditional method of irrigation. Amount of electricity saved for sugarcane under drip was found much more than remaining crops. Electricity consumption to produce one quintal of yield is found significantly less in drip/sprinkler technology as compared to traditional method of irrigation.

5

Role of Government Agencies in Implementation of MIS

An attempt is made in this chapter to describe role of government agencies in promotion of MIS in Maharashtra with special reference to Latur and Osmanabad districts. Results are based on opinions of 40 officers (4 Sub-Divisional Agriculture Officer (SDAO), 18 Taluka Agriculture Officer (TAO), and 18 Circle Agriculture Officer (CAO)) of the selected districts (Table 5.1) Officers are asked to indicate awareness about features of MIS, their role in implementation of MIS, awareness about specific responsibilities, problems, and suggestions for improvement in implementation of MIS.

5.1 Role of Officers

Officers of department of agriculture have important role in promotion, development, and implementation of MIS. As per the guidelines, responsibilities include, among others, creating publicity and awareness among farmers, control and monitoring, acceptance, scrutiny, and sanctioning subsidy proposals, co-ordination with various higher/local departments, training, assessment of water and power, issuance of a/c payee cheques, ensuring after sale services,

Table 5.1
Composition of Officers Interviewed

SN	Officers	District		Total
		Latur	Osmanabad	
1	SDAOs	02	02	04
2	TAOs	10	08	18
3	CAOs	10	08	18
	Total	22	18	40

Source: Field study.

etc. Keeping in view of these roles/responsibilities, an attempt is made in the presents study to assess the awareness of officers about assigned roles/responsibilities, to document the problems faced, and suggestions thereof.

5.2 Awareness of Officers

Officers are asked to indicate their awareness about salient features of MIS (Table 5.2). In all, 5 features are mentioned: water saving, decrease in cost of labour, maximum area allowed under MIS, subsidy, and effective application of fertilizer. Among three categories of officers contacted, SDAOs in both districts are more familiar with the salient features of MIS as compared to TAOs and CAOs. About 91% of the officers (TAOs, and CAOs) in Latur are convinced that MIS contributed in terms of reduction in cost of labour, and savings in water, while it is 100% in Osmanabad. Similarly, 97% of them felt effective application of fertilizer, and maximum area under cultivation is possible through MIS.

Attempts are also made to elicit roles of offices in implementing MIS (Table 5.3). These roles are defined in terms of creating publicity and awareness among farmers, acceptance of proposals, inspection of proposals and forwarding them, selection of farmers, release of subsidy,

Table 5.2
Awareness about Salient Features of MIS

S.N.	Officers	Water Saving	Decrease in Cost of Labour	Maximum Area Allowed	Subsidy	Effective application of fertilizer
(A) Latur						
1	SDAOs	2	2	2	2	2
		(100)	(100)	(100)	(100)	(100)
2	TAOs	10	8	10	10	10
		(100)	(80)	(100)	(100	(100)
3	CAOs	8	10	10	7	9
		(80)	(100)	(100)	(100)	(90)
	Total A	20(91)	20(91)	22(100)	19(80)	21(95)
(B) Osmanabad						
1	SDACs	2	2	2	2	2
		(100)	(100)	(100)	(100)	(100)
2	TAOs	8	7	8	8	8
		(100)	(87)	(100)	(100)	(100)
3	CAOs	8	8	7	8	3
		(100)	(100)	(87)	(100)	(37)
	Total B	18(100)	17(94)	17(94)	18(100)	18(100)
	Grand total (A+B)	38(95)	37(92)	39(97)	37(92)	39(97)

Figures in parentheses are percentages to total officers.
Source: Field study.

Table 5.3
Role of Officers in Implementing MIS

S.N.	Officers	Creating publicity & awareness among farmers	Acceptance of proposals	Inspection of proposals	Forwarding proposals	Selection of farmers	Technical guidance
A. Latur							
1	SDAOs	2 (100)	0	0	0	2 (100)	0
2	TAOs	10 (100)	10 (100)	10 (100)	10 (100)	0	8 (80)
3	CAOs	10 (100)	0	0	0	0	10 (100)
	Total A	22 (100)	10 (45)	10 (45)	10 (45)	2 (2)	18 (82)
B. Osmanabad							
1	SDAOs	2 (100)	0	0	0	2 (100)	0
2	TAOs	8 (100)	8 (100)	8 (100)	8 (100)	8 (100)	0
3	CAOs	8 (100)	8 (100)	0	8 (100)	0	8 (100)
	Total B	18 (100)	16 (89)	8 (44)	16 (89)	10 (56)	8 (44)
	Grand total (A+B)	40 (100)	26 (65)	18 (45)	26 (65)	12 (30)	26 (65)

Figures in parentheses are percentages to total officers.
Source: Field study.

inspection of sets, and to provide technical guidance, if any. Among these issues, creating publicity and awareness among farmers, and sanctioning of proposals are reported by SDAOs. Creating publicity and awareness among farmers, issuing circulars, overall control and monitoring, and sanctioning of proposals are performed by SDAOs. However, SDAOs felt that they don't have any role to perform in acceptance, inspection/scrutiny of farmers' proposals. On the other hand, TAOs reported all activities under consideration, except sanctioning of proposals. CAOs actively participated in creation of publicity, acceptance of proposals, field verifications, and also provided technical guidance to farmers.

Officers are also asked to specify their awareness about specific responsibilities in promotion of MIS (Table 5.4). As agriculture department supplies circulars, and conducts training programmes to its officers, awareness among these officers about their specific responsibilities in promoting MIS is appreciable. In all, 23 responsibilities are mentioned, and they include issuance of circulars and clarifications about MIS, control and monitoring, acceptance of applications, issuing pre-sanction letters, scrutiny of proposals, co-ordination with various higher and local departments, redressal of complaints from farmers and MIS dealers, imposition of penalties against MIS dealers, training, field verification of system design, commissioning of system, field verification of components as per BIS standards, scrutiny and sanctioning of subsidy, ensuring after sale service, and registration of dealers.

Most of the officers are familiar with their responsibilities. Issuance of circulars and making clarification about MIS at district and taluka level is the responsibility of SDAOs (100%), and TAOs (80%) respectively. At the same time, CAOs are involved in field level activities such as field verification of system design, commissioning of the system, drawing samples from field and ensuring after sale services to farmers by MIS service centres.

5.3 Problems

Officers are also asked to mention problems being faced by them in the light of laid guidelines in implementation of MIS at field level (Table 5.5). Officers felt that inadequate electricity supply, lack of awareness among farmers about maintenance of sets, delay in disbursement of subsidy, problems in embossing on sprinkler set, high cost of sand filter, delay in getting grant, and mentioning the name of crops in 7/12 extract of farmers, etc., are the major problems. Vast majority of them reported delays in disbursement of subsidy (93%), and scarcity of electricity as serious challenges in promotion of MIS, and the same need to be attended immediately.

5.4 Suggestions

Suggestions for effective and smooth implementation of MIS based on field level experiences of officers' are given in Table 5.6. They include timely distribution of subsidy, uninterrupted supply of electricity, training to farmers, and availability of grant in time. Officers also mentioned to hike subsidy, and relaxation in requirement of documents from farmers.

5.5 Summary

Roles of government officers, problems faced, and suggestions for improvement in the scheme are covered in this chapter. SDAOs in both districts are more familiar with the salient features of MIS compared to TAOs and CAOs. Majority of officers (TAOs, and CAOs) in both the districts are convinced that MIS contributed in terms of reduction in cost of labour, and savings in water. They felt that effective application of fertilizers and maximum area under cultivation is possible through MIS. Creating publicity and awareness among farmers, issuing circulars, overall control and monitoring, and sanctioning of proposals are performed by SDAOs. CAOs actively participated in verification of design, commissioning

Table 5.4
Awareness about Specific Responsibilities of Officers

S.N.	Responsibilities	A) Latur			Total	B) Osmanabad			Total B	Grand
		SDAO	TAO	CAO	A	SDAO	TAO	CAO		Total (A+B)
1	Issuance of circulars, clarification about MIS	2 (100)	8 (80)	0	10 (45)	2 (10)	8 (100)	8 (100)	18 (100)	28 (70)
2	Control & monitoring	2 (100)	10 (100)	10 (100)	22 (100)	2 (100)	8 (100)	8 (100)	18 (100)	40 (100)
3	Acceptance of applications	1 (50)	10 (100)	0	11 (50)	0	8 (100)	8 (100)	16 (89)	27 (67)
4	Issuing of pre-sanction letters	0	10 (100)	0	10 (45)	2 (100)	8 (100)	0	10 (56)	20 (50)
5	Receiving feasibility report by company	2 (100)	10 (100)	8 (80)	20 (91)	2 (100)	8 (100)	8 (100)	18 (100)	38 (95)
6	Scrutiny of proposal/subsidy	2 (100)	10 (100)	0	12 (55)	2 (100)	8 (100)	8 (100)	18 (100)	30 (75)
7	Co-ordination with various higher/local departments	2 (100)	10 (100)	10 (100)	22 (100)	2 (100)	8 (100)	8 (100)	18 (100)	40 (100)
8	Redressal of complaints from framers, MIS dealers	0	10 (100)	10 (100)	20 (91)	2 (100)	8 (100)	8 (100)	18 (100)	38 (95)

9	Imposition of penalties against MIS dealers	2 (100)	10 (100)	0	12 (55)	2 (100)	0	0	2 (11)	14 (35)
10	Training to farmers	2 (100)	10 (100)	9 (90)	21 (95)	2 (100)	8 (100)	8 (100)	18 (100)	39 (98)
11	Assessment of water and power	2 (100)	0	0	2 (9)	1 (50)	0	0	1 (6)	3 (8)
12	Field verification of system design	2 (100)	5 (50)	10 (100)	17 (77)	0	8 (100)	8 (100)	16 (89)	33 (83)
13	Field verification of commissioning of the system	2 (100)	5 (50)	10 (100)	17 (77)	0	0	8 (100)	8 (44)	25 (63)
14	Field verification of components as per prescribed BIS standards	2 (100)	6 (60)	10 (100)	18 (82)	0	8 (100)	8 (100)	16 (89)	34 (85)
15	Scrutiny of subsidy proposals	2 (100)	10 (100)	0	12 (55)	2 (100)	8 (100)	8 (100)	18 (100)	30 (75)
16	Submission of subsidy proposals for sanction	2 (100)	10 (100)	0	12 (55)	2 (100)	8 (100)	8 (100)	18 (100)	30 (75)
17	Sanction of subsidy proposals	2 (100)	0	0	2 (9)	2 (100)	0	0	2 (11)	4 (10)
18	Issuance of a/c payee cheques to the dealers	2 (100)	0	0	2 (9)	2 (100)	0	0	2 (11)	4 (10)

19	Re-verification of system installation (as per prescribed percentage)	2 (100)	6 (60)	0	8 (36)	0	8 (100)	8 (100)	16 (89)	24 (60)
20	Submission of periodical reports to department	2 (100)	10 (100)	10 (100)	12 (55)	2 (100)	8 (100)	8 (100)	18 (100)	30 (75)
21	Drawing of samples and submission to laboratories	0	0	6 (60)	6 (27)	0	0	8 (100)	8 (44)	14 (35)
22	Ensuring after sale services to the beneficiaries by the MIS service centres	2 (100)	0	10 (100)	12 (55)	2 (100)	8 (100)	8 (100)	18 (100)	30 (75)
23	Registration of dealers	2 (100)	0	0	2 (9)	2 (100)	0	0	2 (11)	4 (10)

Figures in parentheses are percentages to total officers.
Source: Field study.

Table 5.5
Awareness of Officers about Problems in Implementation of the Scheme

S.N.	Responsibilities	A) Latur			Total	B) Osmanabad			Total B	Grand
		SDAO	TAO	CAO	A	SDAO	TAO	CAO		Total (A+B)
1	Inadequate electricity supply	1 (50)	7 (70)	10 (100)	18 (82)	2 (100)	8 (100)	7 (88)	15 (83)	33 (83)
2	Lack of maintenance of the set	0	8 (80)	10 (100)	18 (82)	1 (50)	8 (100)	8 (100)	17 (94)	35 (88)
3	Lack of awareness among farmers about use of system	2 (100)	10 (100)	9 (90)	21 (95)	0	5 (63)	6 (75)	11 (61)	32 (80)
4	Delay in disbursement of subsidy	2 (100)	10 (100)	10 (100)	22 (100)	2 (100)	6 (75)	7 (88)	15 (83)	37 (93)
5	Problem in embossing of name on components of system	1 (50)	9 (90)	8 (80)	18 (82)	2 (100)	8 (100)	8 (100)	18 (83)	36 (93)
6	High cost of sand filter	2 (100)	10 (100)	10 (100)	22 (100)	2 (100)	8 (100)	7 (88)	15 (83)	37 (93)
7	Delay in getting grant	2 (100)	10 (100)	6 (60)	18 (82)	2 (100)	8 (100)	5 (63)	15 (83)	33 (83)
8	Compulsion of mentioning the crop in 7/12 extract	2 (100)	7 (70)	5 (50)	14 (64)	2 (100)	8 (100)	6 (75)	16 (89)	30 (75)

Figures in parentheses are percentages to total officers.
Source: Field study.

Table 5.6

Suggestions Made by Officers for Improvement in the Scheme

S.N.	Suggestions	A) Latur			Total	B) Osmanabad			Total B	Grand Total
		SDAO	TAO	CAO	A	SDAO	TAO	CAO		(A+B)
1	Regular electricity supply	0	10 (100)	10 (100)	20 (91)	2 (100)	8 (100)	7 (88)	17 (94)	37 (93)
2	Regular training to farmers	2 (100)	10 (100)	8 (80)	20 (91)	1 (50)	8 (100)	8 (100)	17 (94)	37 (93)
3	Hike in subsidy	2 (100)	6 (60)	7 (70)	15 (68)	0	5 (63)	6 (75)	11 (61)	26 (65)
4	Embossing of name on components of system	1 (50)	8 (80)	9 (90)	18 (82)	2 (100)	6 (75)	7 (88)	15 (83)	33 (83)
5	Subsidy should be disbursed within two months after installation of system	2 (100)	9 (90)	10 (100)	21 (95)	2 (100)	8 (100)	8 (100)	18 (100)	39 (98)
6	Price list should be available to farmers	2 (100)	7 (70)	8 (80)	17 (77)	2 (100)	8 (100)	7 (88)	17 (94)	34 (85)

7	Grant should be available in time	2 (100)	10 (100)	9 (90)	21 (95)	2 (100)	8 (100)	5 (63)	15 (83)	36 (90)
8	Crop certificate issued by A.O. is sufficient for disbursing the cheque instead of demanding 7/12 document of farmer	2 (100)	10 (100)	8 (80)	20 (91)	2 (100)	8 (100)	6 (75)	16 (89)	36 (90)

Figures in parentheses are percentages to total officers.
Source: Field study.

of the system, drawing samples from field, creation of publicity, and ensuring after sale services to farmers. Officers opined that delay in disbursement of subsidy and scarcity of electricity are the two major problems in promotion of MIS. Officers suggested timely distribution of subsidy, uninterrupted supply of electricity, frequent training to farmers, hike in subsidy, and relaxation in documents required from farmers.

6

Role of Manufacturers in Implementation of MIS

An attempt has been made in this chapter to evaluate the role of MI manufacturers in promoting micro-irrigation in the study area. For this purpose, three frontline enterprises (Jain Irrigation Systems Ltd. (JISL), Plastro Plasson Industries (India) Ltd. (PPIIL), and Exomet Plastics and Chemicals Industries Ltd. (EPCIL)) effectively operational in the study districts and having their headquarters and factory in Maharashtra were selected purposively. The chapter deals with organizational, technical, and quality profiles of the selected manufacturers. Besides this, production, marketing, and promotional activities undertaken by them were also covered. Suggestions for effective and smooth implementation of MIS also formed part of the chapter.

6.1 General Role of MI Manufacturers

MI manufacturers are playing important role in designing, promotion, popularization, extension, and more importantly in horizontal penetration. Apart from quality materials and satisfactory services, price, sustainability and long life of MI system is the key factor for success. Realizing the importance, Government of Maharashtra has been issuing guidelines on do's and don'ts for MI suppliers from time to time. According to the state government, general role to be played by manufacturers in MIS implementation includes promoting the concept of micro-irrigation, supply of BIS standards quality materials, survey, design, supply and install micro-irrigation system as per the standards prescribed, train the farmers regarding maintenance of MI system, provide agronomic support services to the adopters, supply promotional literature in vernacular language (Marathi in Maharashtra), ensure prompt after sales services, facilitates marketing tie ups for the farmer's produce, etc.

6.2 Profiles of MI Manufacturers

A brief profile of selected MI manufacturers is provided in the following sections:

6.2.1 JISL

JISL established in 1987 at Jalgaon district of Maharashtra is a pioneer in MIS in the Indian sub-continent. The firm has multi-product industrial profile and manufactures the full range of precision-irrigation products. According to the official website, JISL is the only manufacturer of complete drip and sprinkler irrigation systems under one roof in the world. JISL is the largest irrigation company in India and stands second globally. Its turnover stood at Rs. 1200 crores in 2006-07. JISL claims to have 50% share in drip irrigation in India.

In addition to drip and sprinkler, JISL also manufactures PVC, polyethylene (HDPE, MDPE), polypropylene piping systems, plastic sheets, dehydrated onions and vegetables, processed fruits, tissue culture, hybrid and grafted plants, greenhouses, poly and shade houses, bio-fertilizers, solar water heating systems and solar photovoltaic appliances, and bio-energy sources. The company renders consultancy for complete or partial project planning and implementation, e.g., watershed and/or crop selection and rotation. JISL has in-house R&D cum demonstration farm at headquarter for showcasing optimum use for best performance of company's hi-tech agricultural inputs and technologies. Company offers training and extension services at their Hi-tech Agri Institute, Jain Hills, Jalgaon. The Institute, besides imparting training to their officials, arranges field visits for government officers, students, scientists, and farmers from all over India as well as from other countries.

Presently the company, besides India, operates in 110 countries of the world with more than 5000 global workforce. State-of-the-art facility of the company got ISO 9001:2000 and 14001:2004 certificates accredited by TUV Germany. With total commitment towards farm and farming community, the company has earned recognition and awards of national and international repute. So far, JISL to its credit has 126 awards for innovative products, 128 for quality aspects, and 2 for export activities.

6.2.2 *PPIIL*

Plastro Plasson Industries (India) Ltd. (PPIIL) is an Indo-Israel joint venture company, established in 1992 and has its registered office at Pune district of Maharashtra. PPIIL offers a wide range of products and solutions in the field of irrigation. PPIIL's services includes survey, planning, and design facilities for drip, mini and micro sprinklers, foggers, misters, fertigation equipments, etc. Solutions offered by the company included tailored drip and micro-irrigation systems, turn-key projects for agriculture sectors such as row crops, horticulture, green house, plantations, orchards, nurseries, etc.

PPIIL is an ISO 9001:2000 company and having technical agreements with world's leading manufacturers. The company has exclusive distributorship for marketing of various irrigation equipments like filters, PVC ball valves, plastic fittings, control valves, automation devices, central control system, etc. Along with its advanced systems, PPIIL also provide comprehensive agronomic guidance and knowledge transfer programmes on irrigation and allied activities. PPIIL has a wide spread network of distributors all over India for sales and services of its products. The company imparts trainings to its stakeholders at their well-equipped training centres located at Pune, Bangalore, Coimbatore, and Delhi.

6.2.3 EPCIL

Exomet Plastics and Chemicals Industry Ltd. (EPCIL) was founded in 1981 as a private limited company and became a public limited company in March 1992. The company is based in Nashik district of Maharashtra. Under MIS production, EPCIL is engaged in drip manufacturing. It also manufactures piping systems for infrastructure gas and water distribution networks, and industry and domestic installations. The manufacturing plant of the company is located at MIDC Ambad, Nashik. The company has branches in Baroda, Bhopal, Coimbatore, Duliajan, Jaipur, Sangli, Thrissur, and Secundrabad. The company imparts training to their officials and farmers at the training centre located in Nashik.

General profiles of manufacturers are provided in Table 6.1. These profiles reveal that all three manufacturers are bonafide, well-equipped, and experienced in their business and comparatively JISL is a giant player.

6.3 Employees with Manufacturers

Qualified, specially trained, and experienced human resource is an asset for any manufacturer. Availability of such resources with manufacturer is important for professional success. In this context, data were collected from select manufacturers and provided in Table 6.2 and 6.3.

Table 6.2 reveals that besides production, manufactures are engaged in various activities like marketing, agri-support and field services, management, administration, R&D, etc.

Table 6.1
Profile of MI Manufacturers

S.N.	Particulars	JISL	PPIIL	EPCIL
1	Registered name	Jain Irrigation Systems Ltd.	Plastro Plasson Industries (India) Ltd.	EPC Industries Ltd.
2	Registration No. and Year	42028 1987	11-067896 1992	L25200MH1981 PLC 025731 1981
3	Form of organisation	Public ltd.	Public ltd.	Public ltd.
4	Location of registered office	Jalgaon (Maharashtra)	Pune (Maharashtra)	Nashik (Maharashtra)
5	Location of head-quarter	Jalgaon (Maharashtra)	Pune (Maharashtra)	Nashik (Maharashtra)
6	Location of marketing office	Jalgaon (Maharashtra)	Pune (Maharashtra)	Nashik (Maharashtra)
7	Location of factory	Jalgaon (Maharashtra)	Pune (Maharashtra)	Nashik (Maharashtra)
8	Location of demo/R&D farms	Jalgaon (Maharashtra)	Pune (Maharashtra)	NA

9	Location of training centres	Jalgaon (Maharashtra)	Pune, Bangalore, Coimbatore, Delhi	Nashik (Maharashtra)
10	Manufacturing	Drip and Sprinkler	Drip	Drip and Sprinkler
11	Manufacturing as	Independent	Joint venture	Independent
12	Tie up with other manufacturer	No	Yes	No
13	Awards and recognitions in irrigation field			
	a) Innovative products	126	1	Nil
	b) Quality	128	Nil	Nil
	c) Export	2	Nil	Nil

Source: Field study.

Table 6.2
Activity-wise Technical Expertise with MI Manufacturers

S.N.	Particulars	JISL	PPIIL	EPCIL
1	Production	1961 (46.23)	34 (11.81)	61 (43.26)
2	Marketing	468 (11.03)	9 (3.12)	8 (5.67)
3	Agri support and field services	235 (5.54)	204 (70.83)	40 (28.37)
4	Management	283 (6.67)	6 (2.08)	2 (1.42)
5	Administration	843 (19.87)	8 (2.78)	8 (5.67)
6	R & D	257 (6.06)	5 (1.74)	3 (2.13)
7	Others	195 (4.60)	22 (7.64)	19 (13.48)
	Total	4242 (100.00)	288 (100.00)	141 (100.00)

Source: Field study.

Table 6.3
Qualification-wise Technical Expertise with MI Manufacturers

S.N.	Particulars	JISL	PPIIL	EPCIL
1	Doctorate	22 (0.52)	1 (0.35)	0
2	Post graduate	444 (10.47)	38 (13.19)	34 (24.11)
3	Graduate	927 (21.85)	144 (50.00)	39 (27.66)
4	Others	2849 (67.16)	105 (36.46)	68 (48.23)
	Total	4242 (100.00)	288 (100.00)	141 (100.00)

Source: Field study.

Obviously, manufactures need diversified personnel like scientists, engineers, technologists, technicians, etc., for smooth and efficient functioning of the company.

Table 6.2 further reveals that JISL has the highest (4242) number of employees followed by PPIIL (288), and EPCIL (141) during 2004-05. Activity-wise, highest percentage of employees of JISL were engaged in production (46.23) followed by administration (19.87), and marketing (11.03). That for PPIIL, it were agri-support and field services (70.83), and production (11.81). In case of EPCIL the corresponding percentages are production (43.26), and agri-support and field services (28.37). Relatively low percentages of employees are working exclusively on R&D in the selected companies.

Qualification-wise break-up of employees with select manufacturers are provided in Table 6.3. Table reveals that JISL and EPCIL have maximum percentages (67.16% and 48.23% respectively) of employees having education below graduation level. In case of PPIIL, about 50% of employees are graduates. The table further reveals that percentage of employees having post graduation are more in case of EPCIL (24.11%) while that of doctorate are found in case of JISL (0.52%).

From above analysis, it could be concluded that JISL compared to others have largest pool of qualified agricultural scientists, technicians, and engineers. Further, quality and quantity of workforce with JISL is significantly on higher side than PPIIL and EPCIL.

6.4 Quality Profiles

Quality of hardware supplied by MI manufacturers is of paramount importance. Poor quality directly affects yield of crops, energy consumption, quantity of water, fertilizers to be delivered to the plant, etc. Besides that durability and life span of component and/or whole system is also reduced. Ultimately this leads to economical losses to the adopter farmers. Quality assurance for MI component/system has been appropriately ensured from MI manufacturers by Government of Maharashtra through guidelines issued from time to time. In this context, the sampled manufacturers were asked for quality parameters and the results are presented in Table 6.4.

Table 6.4 reveals that all three selected manufacturers have ISO series certificates (ISO 9000:140000 (JISL), ISO 9000 (PPIIL), and ISO 9001:2000 (EPCIL)). The MI manufacturers extended one year warranty to the customer-farmers on MI components/system purchased. Quality system practices of JISL and EPCIL is certified by external agency, viz., TUV India and DNV respectively. Components manufactured at respective factories of JISL and EPCIL are tested and approved by external organizations like Central Institute of Plastics Engineering and Technology (CIPET). Quality assurance items mentioned above are reported affirmatively by PPIIL during the interview. However, the details were not provided.

Table 6.4
Quality Profile of MI Manufacturers

SN	Particulars	JISL	PPIIL	EPCIL
1	Type of certification	ISO 9000 : 140000	ISO 9000	ISO 9001: 2000
2	Products covered by warranty	1 year	1 year	1 year
3	Quality system certified by external agency	Yes- TUV India	Yes	Yes- DNV
4	Product tested/ approved by other organization	Yes Central Institute of Plastic Engineering and Technology (CIPET), Mysore	Yes	Yes Central Institute of Plastic Engineering and Technology (CIPET), Mysore

Source: Field study.

Information provided by selected MI manufacturers regarding quality assurance reveals their sincerity towards quality excellence in MIS production.

6.5 Component-wise Manufacturing Status

Guidelines are issued from time to time by Government of Maharashtra to ensure authenticity of manufacturers and quality aspects of MIS. Government expects that manufacturers should have own production capacity of all components. If not, guidelines emphasize minimum production of emitters, emitting pipes, PVC/PE pipes, filtration equipment and fertigation equipment in case of drip manufacturing. As of sprinkler manufacturers, sprinkler heads/nozzles, fittings, and polyethylene pipes are to be produced. Rest of the components may be procured from outside but without compromising prescribed quality and specification. With this backdrop, selected manufacturers were asked to supply production status of the components of both drip and sprinkler irrigation system. The results are provided in Table 6.5.

It could be observed from the table that except JISL, PPIIL and EPCIL procured one or another component of either drip or sprinkler irrigation system from outside agency. PPIIL procured components namely HDPE pipes, HDPE pipe fittings, and screen filter for drip irrigation system, and QRC sprinkler pipe, QRC fittings, and sprinklers (nozzles) for sprinkler irrigation system. While EPCIL procured poly fittings, PVC pipes, PVC fittings, and disc filters for drip irrigation system and rainguns, PVC ball valves, GM valves, air release valves, non-return valves, and GI fittings for sprinkler irrigation system. Rest of the components under consideration is manufactured by PPIIL and EPCIL at their respective factories.

6.6 Sales Network

As a part of business, manufacturers establish sales offices and deploy their sales staff at important locations. They also create network of dealers at village, taluka and/or district/ division level to ensure maximum customer coverage and prompt after sales services. Sampled MI manufacturers were

Table 6.5
Components Manufactured/Procured by MI Manufacturers

S.N.	Item	JISL		PPIIL		EPCIL	
		Self	Pro-cured	Self	Pro-cured	Self	Pro-cured
1	Drippers/Emitters NPC	√	–	√	–	√	–
2	Drippers/Emitters PC	√	–	√	–	–	–
3	Emitting pipes/ inline drip laterals	√	–	√	–	√	–
4	Poly laterals	√	–	√	–	√	–
5	Poly fittings	√	–	√	–	–	√
6	PVC pipes	√	–	√	–	–	√
7	PVC fittings	√	–	√	–	–	√
8	HDPE pipes	√	–	–	√	√	–
9	HDPE pipe fittings	√	–	–	√	√	–
10	Screen filters	√	–	√	√	√	–
11	Disc filters	√	–	√	–	–	√
12	Media (sand) filters	√	–	√	–	√	–
13	Hydrocyclone/ sand separator	√	–	–	–	√	–
14	QRC sprinkler pipe	√	–	–	√	√	–
15	QRC fittings	√	–	–	√	√	–
16	Sprinklers (Nozzle)	√	–	–	√	√	–
17	Rainguns	√	–	–	–	–	√
18	PVC ball valves	√	–	–	–	–	√
19	GM valves	√	–	–	–	–	√
20	Air release valves	√	–	–	–	–	√
21	Non-return valves	√	–	–	–	–	√
22	GI fittings	√	–	–	–	–	√

Source: Field study.

asked to supply information for their sales network at state level as well as in study districts (Table 6.6).

Items under consideration like number of dealers/ distributors, number of sales staff, and number of regional offices during 2007-08 at state level were reported on higher side (650, 71, and 14 respectively) for JISL. On the other hand, number of survey and installation agencies, and number

Table 6.6
Sales Network of MI Manufacturers

SN	Particulars	JISL	PPIIL	EPCIL
Latur				
1	No. of regional offices	1	0	0
2	No. of sales offices	1	1	0
3	No. of sales staff	1	1	4
4	No. of dealers/distributors	17	3	5
5	No. of survey & installation agencies	2	2	0
Osmanabad				
1	No. of regional offices	0	1	0
2	No. of sales offices	0	1	0
3	No. of sales staff	0	1	2
4	No. of dealers/distributors	13	5	5
5	No. of survey & installation agencies	2	5	0
Maharashtra				
1	No. of regional offices	14	4	1
2	No. of sales offices	14	20	2
3	No. of sales staff	71	20	13
4	No. of dealers/distributors	650	189	90
5	No. of survey & installation agencies	20	50	0

Source: Field study.

of sales offices were found more (50 and 14 respectively) in PPIIL.

Strength of sales staff in EPCIL (4) and number of dealers/ distributors in JISL (17) were reported on higher side in Latur district, while number of survey and installation agencies were reported higher for PPIIL (5) in Osmanabad district. JISL has its regional office and sales office in Latur district only while EPCIL has no regional/sales office in both the districts.

6.7 Sales Performance

Sales turnover is a thermometer of business for any manufacturer which in turn indicates the financial health. Abnormal ups and downs in sales warrants appropriate strategies by the manufacturer. Considering the importance of sales turnover, data obtained in this regard from select manufacturers are provided in Table 6.7.

It is discernable from Table 6.7 that sale of drip sets by JISL is more than sprinkler sets, and also more than drip sets than that of PPIIL in Maharashtra during 2001-05. Further, sales of drip and sprinkler sets by JISL and PPIIL reported significant decline during the period under consideration. JISL reported highest (Rs. 5513.94 lakhs) sale of drip sets during 2000-01 which declined to Rs. 3780.01 lakhs in 2004-05. That for sprinkler set the corresponding figures are Rs. 1593.20 lakhs in 2000-01 and Rs. 1076.97 lakhs in 2004-05. Sale of drip sets by PPIIL also declined from Rs. 899.93 lakhs in 2000-01 to Rs. 780.50 lakhs in 2004-05.

JISL reported highest (Rs. 322.35 lakhs) sale of drip sets in Osmanabad during 2001-02 and that of Rs. 142.01 lakhs for sprinkler sets in Latur during 2004-05. Except 2003-04 and 2004-05 in Latur, sale of drip sets in both the districts were reported to be on higher side than that of sprinkler sets. By and large, sale of drip and sprinkler sets of JISL in Latur reported upward trend from 2002-03 to 2004-05 whereas declining trend was noticed in Osmanabad. PPIIL has been selling only drip sets and exhibited mixed trend in both the districts. Information regarding sale of both the items by EPCIL were not provided.

6.8 Promotional Activities

Besides supply of quality MI equipments, manufactures are expected to extend various support services. Idea behind providing these services is to harness the benefit of MI technology to the ultimate beneficiary-farmers. Various promotional activities undertaken by the sampled manufacturers are provided in Table 6.8.

Promotional activities like supply of comprehensive produce catalogue for all manufactured products, O&M manual in Marathi, crop booklets describing adoption of micro-irrigation based on Indian experience, literature in Marathi, trainings to MI adopters, after sales services, and general maintenance services to adopters are being undertaken by all three MI manufacturers. However, activity like comprehensive product catalogue for all OEM/procured products were not undertaken by PPIIL and EPCIL. Further, agronomic and marketing services were also not provided by EPCIL and PPIIL. Thus, it is noteworthy to mention here that JISL is providing all the promotional activities under consideration to the beneficiary-farmers.

6.9 Suggestions for Improvement

Following suggestions were provided by the manufacturers for effective implementation of MIS.

6.9.1 JISL

1. Paper work related to the subsidy proposals and spot assessment need to be reduced. Movement of subsidy proposal should be from AO → TAO → SAO → TAO → disbursal to the beneficiary (Farmer/Company/Bank).
2. As far as possible payment should be made within 30 days after commissioning the system so as to take care of the interests of both farmers and manufacturers.
3. If there is a delay of more than 8 days from TAO, the proposal must be treated as deemed to be confirmed.
4. Advance subsidy may be given to the manufacturer for lateral, etc., against the bank guarantee extended by the company.
5. Registration of any company must be allowed only and only if they are manufacturing minimum five parts as follows: (i) Lateral, (ii) Dripper, (iii) Inline, (iv) PVC Pipes, and (v) Filter.
6. If farmer failed to continue to utilize the set at least for three years in a working condition, 50% subsidy should be recovered after verification.

Table 6.7
Sales Performance (Rs. lakhs) of MI Manufacturers

S.N.	Year	JISL		PPIIL		EPCIL	
		Drip	Sprin.	Drip	Sprin.	Drip	Sprin.
Latur							
1	2000-01	75.55 (1.37)	72.99 (4.58)	2.17 (0.24)	NA	NP	NP
2	2001-02	235.48 (4.56)	97.6 (9.74)	0	NA	NP	NP
3	2002-03	25.76 (0.86)	4.95 (1.53)	0	NA	NP	NP
4	2003-04	48.18 (1.32)	58.38 (7.76)	0.24 (0.04)	NA	NP	NP
5	2004-05	52.47 (1.39)	142.01 (13.19)	7.85 (1.00)	NA	NP	NP
Osmanabad							
1	2000-01	77.2 (1.40)	18.43 (1.16)	322.65 (35.85)	NA	NP	NP
2	2001-02	322.35 (6.24)	9.66 (0.96)	531.25 (47.23)	NA	NP	NP
3	2002-03	41.96 (1.41)	1.36 (0.42)	12.87 (2.42)	NA	NP	NP

4	2003-04	34.4 (0.94)	11.93 (1.58)	1.42 (0.27)	NA	NP	NP
5	2004-05	28.45 (0.75)	11.01 (1.02)	11.43 (1.46)	NA	NP	NP
Maharashtra							
1	2000-01	5513.94 (100.00)	1593.2 (100.00)	899.93 (100.00)	NA	NP	NP
2	2001-02	5167.07 (100.00)	1002.26 (100.00)	1124.86 (100.00)	NA	NP	NP
3	2002-03	2976.62 (100.00)	323.1 (100.00)	532.61 (100.00)	NA	NP	NP
4	2003-04	3658.02 (100.00)	752.04 (100.00)	531.27 (100.00)	NA	NP	NP
5	2004-05	3780.01 (100.00)	1076.97 (100.00)	780.5 (100.00)	NA	NP	NP

Source: Field study.
NA = Not applicable; NP = Not provided

Table 6.8
Promotional Activities Undertaken by MI Manufacturers

S.N.	Activity	JISL	PPIIL	EPCIL
1	Comprehensive product catalogue for all manufactured products	Yes	Yes	Yes
2	Comprehensive product catalogue for all OEM/procured products	Yes	No	No
3	Operation and maintenance manual in Marathi	Yes	Yes	Yes
4	Crop booklets describing adoption of micro-irrigation based on Indian experience	Yes	Yes	Yes
5	Promotional literature in Marathi	Yes	Yes	Yes
6	Training to MI adopters	Yes	Yes	Yes
7	After sales service	Yes	Yes	Yes
8	Agronomic services to adopters	Yes	Yes	No
9	Marketing services to adopters	Yes	No	Yes
10	General maintenance services to adopters	Yes	Yes	Yes

Source: Field study.

7. Compulsory training and service camps should be organized in collaboration with State Agriculture Universities.
8. State government should release subsidy without waiting for centre's share.

6.9.2 PPIIL

1. MSMIP in project format is to be implemented on the lines of Andhra Pradesh Micro Irrigation Project (APMIP) and Gujarat Micro Irrigation Project (GMIP) on an urgent basis.
2. Monitoring of MIS implementation in the state be undertaken jointly with all certified MI manufacturing companies, state government, and farmers' representatives.
3. Subsidy to the beneficiary-farmers must be released within one month form the date of installation.

6.9.3 EPCIL

1. Fresh relook is required into the subject of subsidy component of the MIS implementation.
2. MSMIP should be implemented on the lines of APMIP and GMIP.
3. Monitoring of MI implementation should be made strict.
4. Adoption of drip/sprinkler should be made mandatory along with subsidy to all farmers cultivating sugarcane, orchards, etc.

6.10 Summary

Role of manufacturers is studied in this chapter. All three MI manufacturers are bonafide, well-equipped, and experienced. JISL is a giant player in MIS production, and has largest pool of qualified agricultural scientists, technicians, and engineers. Further, quality and quantity of workforce with JISL is significantly on higher side than PPIIL and EPCIL. Information provided by selected manufacturers regarding quality assurance revealed their sincerity towards quality. Except JISL, PPIIL and EPCIL procured one or another component of either drip or sprinkler irrigation system from outside. Number of dealers/distributors, number of sales staff, and number of regional offices at state level were reported on higher side for JISL than PPIIL and EPCIL. JISL has its regional/sales office in Latur only while EPCIL has neither regional office nor sales office in the study area. Sales of drip and sprinkler sets by JISL and PPIIL reported significant decline during the period under consideration. Suggestions for effective implementation of MIS included prompt release of subsidy, confirmation of subsidy proposal within specific time period, minimum component production criteria, extensive training programmes to farmers, implementation of MSMIP on the lines of APMIP and GMIP, strict and joint monitoring, etc. In nutshell, besides supplying BIS standard quality materials and support services to the adopters, manufacturers have been playing important role in promotion, popularization, extension, and more importantly, in horizontal penetration of MIS in the study area.

7
Role of Dealers in Implementation of MIS

Role of dealers in promotion of MIS in selected districts is covered in this chapter. It deals with analysis of basic information on dealers, average sets marketed, financial performance, awareness about their responsibilities in promotion of MIS, training programmes conducted, problems faced, and suggestions for improvement.

7.1 Role of Dealers

MIS dealers are assigned with important activities in promotion of micro-irrigation scheme. As per the guidelines of the state government, they are to promote and popularize the concept of micro-irrigation, survey, design, supply and install micro-irrigation systems as per prescribed standards, provide agronomy services, facilitate marketing tie-ups for the farmers' produce, train the farmers regarding maintenance of micro-irrigation systems, provide after sale services, and supply BIS standard and quality material. Dealer should have a qualified engineer from company. Survey of farmer's land and collection of relevant data base are also the responsibilities of the dealer. Keeping in view of these important roles, an attempt is made to assess their awareness, problems faced, and suggestions for further improvement in implementation.

7.2 Dealers' Awareness

In all, 8 dealers (Table 7.1) are selected from Latur and Osmanabad districts representing NOCIL, Hasti, Netafim, Jain, Rungta, Nagarjuna, EPC, Plastro Plasson Industries, and Das. Among these dealers, 4 passed professional (technical) degrees (BE, MSc., and BSc.), 2 studied up to B.A., and the rest completed HSC. The year of registration of dealership ranged from 1984 to 2002. Keerti agency in Latur district is oldest dealer, while Rajesh Krishi Seva Kendra in Osmanabad is registered in 2002.

Both drip and sprinkler sets marketed by dealers, and their financial performance is provided in Appendices 7.1 to 7.4. Average sets of drip and sprinklers marketed by these dealers during 2000-01 to 2004-05 are depicted in Table 7.2. As observed from the table, sale of sprinkler sets is more in Latur district as compared to Osmanabad, while sale of drip sets is higher in Osmanabad. Average sale of drip and sprinklers ranged from 285 to 573, and 73 to 218 respectively during 2000-01 to 2004-05.

Financial performance is provided in Table 7.3. The average price per set of drip ranged from Rs. 0.42 lakh to 0.43 lakh, and that of sprinkler from Rs. 0.18 lakh to Rs. 0.20 lakh. The average amount of sale of drip sets ranged from Rs. 119.49 lakhs to Rs. 243.31 lakhs, but in the case of sprinkler sets it was Rs. 13.14 lakhs to Rs. 43.00 lakhs. As the sale of drip sets in Osmanabad is more than that of Latur, total value of sale is also higher.

Dealers selected for the study in Latur and Osmanabad districts are asked to inform their awareness on responsibilities in promotion of MIS (Table 7.4). Responsibilities of MIS dealers are defined in terms of availability of system design engineer, conduct of survey of fields before installation of MIS, testing of soil and water, design of MIS, supply of BIS

Table 7.1
Details of Dealers Interviewed

S.N.	Name	Education	Year of Registration	Name of the Company	Type of Set
A. Latur					
1	Keerti Agencies	B.E.	1984	NOCIL, Hasti	Sprinkler
2	Padmini Agencies	B.A.	1997	Netafim	Drip
3	Mahalaxmi Drip & Sprinkler Agencies	B.Sc.	1999	Jain & Rungta	Drip, Sprinkler
4	Shri Sainath Agro agencies	HSC	1998	Nagarjuna, EPC	Drip, Sprinkler
B. Osmanabad					
1	Rajesh Krishi Seva Kendra	7th	2002	Jain	Drip, Sprinkler
2	Amol Agency	M.Sc.	1995	Plastro Plasson Industries (India) Ltd.	Drip
3	Shree Shaneshwar Agro Services	B.A.	2001	DAS	Drip
4	Mohiniraj Irrigation Service	B.Sc.	1999	EPC	Drip, Sprinkler

Source: Field study.

Table 7.2
Average Sets Marketed by Sample Dealers

S.N.	Years	Latur		Osmanabad		Average	
		Drip	Sprinkler	Drip	Sprinkler	Drip	Sprinkler
1	2000-01	64	136	505	10	285	73
2	2001-02	90	141	1040	15	565	78
3	2002-03	87	404	1058	32	573	218
4	2003-04	96	292	580	35	338	164
5	2004-05	100	415	494	15	297	215

Source: Field study.

Table 7.3
Average Financial Performance (Rs. lakhs) of Sample Dealers

S.N.	Years	Latur		Osmanabad		Average	
		Drip	Sprinkler	Drip	Sprinkler	Drip	Sprinkler
1	2000-01	26.88	24.48	212.10	1.80	119.49	13.14
2	2001-02	37.80	25.38	436.80	2.70	237.30	14.04
3	2002-03	36.97	76.76	449.65	6.08	243.31	41.42
4	2003-04	41.28	58.40	249.40	7.00	145.34	32.70
5	2004-05	43.00	83.00	212.42	3.00	127.71	43.00

Source: Field study.

standard materials, to provide after sale service, visit of engineer to farmer's field, charges made for installation of MIS, supply of post cards, complaints received by post-cards, providing booklets on operation and maintenance of system, and crop manuals to the beneficiary. Dealers are aware of most of the responsibilities. Out of eight, three in Latur and one in Osmanabad reported testing of water and soil undertaken before designing the system. None of them reported sale of non-BIS standard materials, and at the same time no charge was levied on secondary transportation to farmer's field. One dealer informed charging for spare parts during warranty period. Dealers also reported about receiving complaints by post-cards, which were attended promptly.

Conducting training in the field of MIS is one of the important activities undertaken by dealers. Status of training programmes conducted by dealers in study area is given in Table 7.5. Field demonstration, visit to successful plots of MIS, farmers' fair (Shetkari Melava), and organization of exhibitions of MIS are main activities covered. Average number of farmers trained was 5332, and incurred amount of Rs. 0.90 lakhs, companies contributed 50% of the total expenditure on training.

7.3 Problems

Problems faced by dealers in selected districts are given in Table 7.6. They include additional expenditure and cumbersome procedure involved in elaborate embossing on all spare parts including minor ones, incorrect technical specification of sprinkler set by government department, lack of finance, undue delay in verification of farmers' documents, farmers unwillingness to buy sand filter, and lack of technical knowledge on the part of farmer.

7.4 Suggestions

Opinions of dealers and their suggestions for effective implementation are explained in Table 7.7. Most of the dealers

Table 7.4

Awareness of Dealers about Their Responsibilities in MIS

S.N.	Responsibilities	District		Average
		Latur	Osmanabad	
1	Availability of MIS system design engineer	4	4	4
2	Engineer deputed by the company	4	3	4
3	Qualified engineer	4	4	4
4	Conduct of survey of fields before installation of MIS	3	4	4
5	Testing of water & soil undertaken before designing the system	3	1	2
6	Design of MIS prepared before installation	3	4	3
7	Supply BIS standard material	4	4	4
8	Supply non-BIS standard material	0	0	0
9	To provide after sale service	4	4	4
10	Visit of engineer to the farmers' field	4	4	4
11	Charge for installation of MIS at farmers' fields	2	4	3
12	Charge for secondary transportation to the farmers' field	0	0	0
13	Sale/supply on credit	2	1	2
14	Other charges levied for MIS in the bill	0	0	0
15	Helping farmers in preparation and submission of subsidy proposals	4	4	4
16	Liasioning with agricultural department	4	4	4

17	Imparting training to beneficiaries-farmers in operation and management of system	4	4	4
18	Providing literature on operation and management of system	4	4	4
19	Providing literature on package of practices for different crops	3	4	3
20	Training from manufacturers	4	4	4
21	Charge for spares during warranty	1	0	1
22	Warranty for system components	4	3	3
23	Samples drawn from your premises failed in test so far	0	0	0
24	Initiatives taken for promotion of the scheme	4	4	4
25	*Modus operendi* of sales promotion/convincing farmers	4	4	4
26	Any other monetary incentives offered to farmers	2	2	2
27	Supply post-cards, service coupons to farmers	4	4	4
28	Attending the complaints received by post-cards	4	4	4
29	Providing mandatory free services to farmers as per coupon system provided in guidelines of Agril. Dept.	4	4	4
30	Financial incentives from manufacturer for sale	4	2	3
31	Providing booklets on operation and maintenance of system, crop manuals to the beneficiary farmers	4	4	4

Source: Field study.

Table 7.5
Status of Training Programmes Conducted by Selected dealers

S.N.	District	Farmer's Trained	Cost of Training (Rs. lakhs)	Contribution by Company (Rs. lakhs)
1	Latur	6665	1.38	0.69
2	Osmanabad	4000	0.42	0.21
	Average	5332	0.90	0.45

Source: Field study.

Table 7.6
Awareness of Dealers about Problems Faced in MIS

S.N.	Problems	District		Average
		Latur	Osmanabad	
1	Embossing all information on spare parts of sets	02	03	3
2	Farmer purchases only pipes not nozzles	00	04	2
3	Delay in disbursement of subsidy	04	04	4
4	Load shedding (electricity)	04	04	4
5	Non-availability of technical/design engineers in Govt. department	01	03	2
6	Technical specification of sprinkler set given by Dept. is not correct (Number of nozzles and length of pipe)	0	03	1
7	Lack of finance	04	04	4
8	Undue delay in verification of farmer's documents	03	04	3
9	Farmer does not buy sand filter	04	04	4
10	Lack of technical knowledge of farmer	04	04	4

Source: Field study.

Table 7.7
Suggestions Provided by Dealers for Improvement in MIS

S.N.	Problems	District		Average
		Latur	Osmanabad	
1	Subsidy should be based on market price of the set.	04	04	4
2	Quick verification of farmer's documents.	03	04	3
3	Use of sprinkler set should not be for specified crops.	04	04	4
4	Specification of number of nozzles per pipe should be increased from 5 to 10.	00	03	1
5	Sand filter must be included under subsidy.	04	04	4
6	MIS should be implemented on the line of A.P. and Gujarat states.	04	04	4
7	Company should give sales incentives to dealers.	04	04	4
8	Norms of Government should not change frequently.	04	04	4
9	Department should arrange workshop for farmers to understand technical knowledge of set.	04	04	4
10	Farmers should be supported by sufficient finance.	04	04	4

Source: Field study.

suggested to fix subsidy on the basis of market price, allow use of sprinkler for all crops, to include cost of sand filter in subsidy, implementation of MIS on the lines of Andhra Pradesh and Gujarat's Micro Irrigation Project, sales incentives to dealers by companies, consistency in government's guidelines, arranging workshops, visits, etc., for farmers. Last but not the least, providing sufficient financial assistance to farmers to purchase MIS set with all spare parts.

7.5 Summary

This chapter is aimed at examining role of dealers in the implementation of MIS. Out of eight dealers studied, six dealers were studied up to graduation and postgraduation. More number of drip sets were sold in Osmanabad (505) compared to Latur (64) in 2000-01, and it was 494 and 100 respectively during 2004-05. Invariably, cost of drip is more than sprinkler set. More farmers were trained in Latur (6665) than in Osmanabad (4000). Most of the dealers suggested to fix subsidy on market price, and also to include cost of sand filter. They were not getting incentives on sales from companies, hence were unhappy. Dealers also complained about additional expenditure and cumbersome procedure involved in elaborate embossing on all spare parts including minor ones. Dealers further suggested allowing use of sprinkler for all crops, implementation of MIS on the lines of Andhra Pradesh and Gujarat's Micro Irrigation Project, consistency in government's guidelines, and arranging workshops, visits, etc., for farmers.

8

Farmers' Feedback on Micro-irrigation System

Chapters 3 and 4 established positive relationship between drip/sprinkler technology and crop productivity and reduction in input costs. An attempt is made in the chapter to highlight the problems faced and future prospects of MIS in the study area.

8.1 Problems Faced by Sample Farmers

Sample farmers were interviewed to probe into various financial, operational, quality aspects, and marketing problems in order to suggest measures to overcome the same. Findings are presented in Table 8.1.

Table 8.1 revealed that all farmers using drip/sprinkler technology faced frequent load shedding and hence felt handicapped in efficient utilization of various inputs. High initial costs, delay in subsidy, poor technical assistance from manufactures, lack of remunerative price, high operation and maintenance costs, poor technical assistance from government agency, and frequent chocking of system (93%, 89%, 81%, 77%, 72%, 72%, and 70% respectively) were reported by drip adopters. Though relative percentages slightly varied, similar

Table 8.1
Problems Faced by Farmers Using MIS

S.N.	Problem	Latur					
		Drip (n= 136)			Sprinkler (n= 224)		
		Yes	No	Don't know	Yes	No	Don't know
1	In getting subsidy	115 (84.56)	21 (15.44)	-	181 (80.80)	43 (19.20)	-
2	Bank takes long time for sanction	72 (52.94)	38 (27.94)	26 (19.12)	87 (38.84)	101 (45.09)	36 (16.07)
3	High initial cost	127 (93.38)	9 (6.62)	-	116 (51.79)	108 (48.21)	-
4	Frequent choking/other problems with the system	89 (65.44)	47 (34.56)	-	22 (9.82)	202 (90.18)	-
5	Frequent load shedding	136 (100.00)	-	-	224 (100.00)	-	-
6	Operation and maintenance cost is high	93 (68.38)	43 (31.62)	-	29 (12.95)	195 (87.05)	-
7	Temporary or permanent failure of system	30 (22.06)	106 (77.94)	-	27 (12.05)	197 (87.95)	-
8	Material quality of equipment is not good	68 (50.00)	51 (37.50)	17 (12.50)	16 (7.14)	200 (89.29)	8 (3.57)
9	Poor technical assistance from manufacturer	98 (72.06)	38 (27.94)	-	144 (64.29)	80 (35.71)	-

10	Poor technical assistance from government agency	111 (81.62)	25 (18.38)	-	173 (77.23)	51 (22.77)	-
11	Occurrence of new disease and pest	-	107 (78.68)	29 (21.32)	-	212 (94.64)	12 (5.36)
12	Spare parts not available in time	47 (34.56)	89 (65.44)	-	7 (3.12)	217 (96.88)	-
13	Lack of marketing facilities	42 (30.88)	94 (69.12)	-	25 (11.16)	199 (88.84)	-
14	Lack of remunerative prices	89 (65.44)	47 (34.56)	-	173 (77.23)	51 (22.77)	-
15	Lack of storage facility	55 (40.44)	81 (59.56)	-	108 (48.21)	116 (51.79)	-
16	Others	34 (25.00)	102 (75.00)	-	10 (4.46)	214 (95.54)	-

Table 8.1 Contd...

S.N.	Problem	Latur					
		Drip (n= 507)			Sprinkler (n= 53)		
		Yes	No	Don't know	Yes	No	Don't know
1	In getting subsidy	455 (89.74)	52 (10.26)	-	38 (71.70)	15 (28.30)	-
2	Bank takes long time for sanction	338 (66.67)	135 (26.63)	34 (6.70)	29 (54.72)	16 (30.18)	8 (15.10)
3	High initial cost	470 (92.70)	37 (7.30)	-	31 (58.49)	22 (41.51)	-
4	Frequent choking/other problems with the system	361 (71.20)	146 (28.80)	-	13 (24.53)	40 (75.47)	-
5	Frequent load shedding	507 (100.00)	-	-	53 (100.00)	-	-
6	Operation and maintenance cost is high	372 (73.37)	135 (26.63)	-	18 (33.96)	35 (66.04)	-
7	Temporary or permanent failure of system	327 (64.50)	166 (32.74)	14 (2.76)	8 (15.10)	45 (84.90)	-
8	Material quality of equipment is not good	306 (60.36)	140 (27.61)	61 (12.03)	10 (18.87)	43 (81.13)	-
9	Poor technical assistance from manufacturer	422 (83.23)	85 (16.77)	-	34 (64.15)	19 (35.85)	-

10	Poor technical assistance from government agency	354 (69.82)	153 (30.18)	-	32 (60.38)	21 (39.62)	-
11	Occurrence of new disease and pest	-	318 (62.72)	189 (37.28)	-	36 (67.92)	17 (32.08)
12	Spare parts not available in time	321 (63.31)	186 (36.69)	-	14 (26.42)	39 (73.58)	-
13	Lack of marketing facilities	169 (33.33)	338 (66.67)	-	17 (32.08)	36 (67.92)	-
14	Lack of remunerative prices	409 (80.67)	98 (19.33)	-	35 (66.04)	18 (33.96)	-
15	Lack of storage facility	219 (43.20)	288 (56.80)	-	24 (45.28)	29 (54.72)	-
16	Others	389 (76.73)	118 (23.27)	-	12 (22.64)	41 (77.36)	-

Table 8.1 contd...

S.N.	Problem	Osmanabad					
		Drip (n=507)			Sprinkler (n= 53)		
		Yes	No	Don't know	Yes	No	Don't know
1	In getting subsidy	570 (88.65	73 (11.35)	-	219 (79.06)	58 (20.94)	-
2	Bank takes long time for sanction	410 (63.76)	173 (26.91)	60 (9.33)	116 (41.88)	117 (42.24)	44 (15.88)
3	High initial cost	597 (92.85)	46 (7.15)	-	147 (53.07)	130 (46.93)	-
4	Frequent choking/other problems with the system	450 (69.98)	193 (30.02)	-	35 (12.64)	242 (87.36)	-
5	Frequent load shedding	643 (100.00)	-	-	277 (100.00)	-	-
6	Operation and maintenance cost is high	465 (72.32)	178 (27.68)	-	47 (16.97)	230 (83.03)	-
7	Temporary or permanent failure of system	357 (55.52)	272 (42.30)	14 (2.18)	35 (12.64)	242 (87.36)	-
8	Material quality of equipment is not good	374 (58.16)	191 (29.71)	78 (12.13)	26 (9.39)	243 (87.73)	8 (2.88)
9	Poor technical assistance from manufacturer	520 (80.87)	123 (19.13)	-	178 (64.26)	99 (35.74)	-
10	Poor technical assistance from government agency	465 (72.32	178 (27.68)	-	205 (74	72 (26.00)	-

11	Occurrence of new disease and pest	-	425 (66.10)	218 (33.90)	-	248 (89.53)	29 (10.47)
12	Spare parts not available in time	368 (57.23)	275 (42.77)	-	21 (7.58)	256 (92.42)	-
13	Lack of marketing facilities	211 (32.81)	432 (67.19)	-	42 (15.16)	235 (84.84)	-
14	Lack of remunerative prices	498 (77.45)	145 (22.55)	-	208 (75.10)	69 (24.90)	-
15	Lack of storage facility	274 (42.61)	369 (57.39)	-	132 (47.65)	145 (52.35)	-
16	Others	423 (65.79)	220 (34.21)	-	22 (7.94)	255 (92.06)	-

Figures in brackets indicate percentage to the respective sample size.
Source : Field study.

problems were also reported by sprinkler adopters. Spread of new pests and diseases due to MIS adoption was not noticed by the farmers.

More or less, similar pattern was noticed in both the districts. Across technologies, problems like high initial costs, frequent chocking, poor quality material, and non-availability of spare parts in time were found much severe for drip adopters compared to sprinkler adopters. Owing to high initial capital cost of drip, sample farmers tempted to by-pass sand filter in order to keep the cost in their reach. High PH and physical impurities in irrigation water lead to frequent chocking of set and reduced overall efficiency. Poor quality material of drip set further increased the severity. Chocking of nozzles and cracking of laterals occurred frequently in drip set and hence needed replacements. Time lag between obtaining these spare parts from dealers located at district places and replacing the same significantly affected the valuable crop besides increased additional cost for sample farmers. Because of frequent chocking and cracking coupled with biological accidents (cuts by rat/rodents and roots growth in nozzles) lead to temporary or permanent failure of the system, more often in drip. This also increased operation and maintenance cost significantly for drip adopters.

Respondents expected frequent technical assistance from manufacturer/dealers and government agency. Unfortunately, despite legal bindings on service providers and facilitators to provide such services, the same were found unsatisfactory and warrants immediate correction. Delay in subsidy disbursement and amount of subsidy (50% of capital cost or upper ceiling limit in rupees per acre) in the context of market price greatly disappointed respondents. Recognizing the high capital cost and need for adoption of these technologies, provision for bank loan has been made. Critical loaning procedure and requirement of number of papers consumed valuable time and money. Necessary policy measures based on realistic approach is must to maintain orderliness and greater diffusion of these technologies.

8.2 Farmers' Satisfaction

Farmers availing services of drip/sprinkler technology in the study districts subject to numerous financial, technical, and administrative problems. Considering this, an attempt has been made to know the satisfaction of sample farmers. Results are presented in Table 8.2.

Table 8.2 reveals that majority (75% to 85%) of farmers were not satisfied with the present after sale services provided, and training and visits given by dealers and government officers. Ultimately, about 60% drip adopters at overall level were found dissatisfied about the working of the system. Major reasons behind this were substandard material, cracking of laterals, chocking of nozzles, and high operation and maintenance cost. Comparatively about 91% sprinkler adopters were found satisfied about the working of sprinkler system.

Drip/sprinkler adopters of Latur were found more satisfied than Osmanabad. Higher percentages of farmers were satisfied with sprinkler than drip. Respondents were dissatisfied with after sale services, training programmes, and visits by dealers/government officers. Comparatively, higher percentages of farmers from Latur were satisfied with the above services.

It could be concluded that the farmers cultivating cash crops under capital intensive MIS needed trouble-free and quality sets for efficient working of the system on prolonged basis. Technical aspects involved in these technologies warrants prompt after sale services, need-based trainings, and regular visits by service providers and facilitators.

8.3 Farmers' Willingness towards Future Expansion of Area under MIS

Willingness of farmers to extend area under drip/sprinkler is determined by performance of these technologies at farm level. Considering this, sample farmers were interviewed

Table 8.2
Satisfaction Level of Farmers

S.N.	Particulars	Category		Latur No.	Latur %	Osmanabad No.	Osmanabad %	Total No.	Total %
1	Working of system	a) Drip	i) Yes	77	56.62	179	35.3	256	39.81
			ii) No	59	43.38	328	64.7	387	60.19
		b) Sprinkler	i) Yes	210	93.75	43	81.13	253	91.34
			ii) No	14	6.25	10	18.87	24	8.66
2	After sale services		a) Yes	112	31.11	114	20.36	226	24.57
			b) No	248	68.89	446	79.64	694	75.43
3	Training by dealers		a) Yes	101	28.06	177	31.61	278	30.22
			b) No	259	71.94	383	68.39	642	69.78
4	Training by government officers		a) Yes	89	24.72	109	19.46	198	21.52
			b) No	271	75.28	451	80.54	722	78.48
5	Visits by dealers		a) Yes	56	15.56	74	13.21	130	14.13
			b) No	304	84.44	486	86.79	790	85.87
6	Visits by government officers		a) Yes	84	23.23	94	16.79	178	19.35
			b) No	276	76.67	466	83.21	742	80.65

Source : Field study.

and results are presented in Table 8.3. Interestingly, about 85% sample farmers expressed their willingness for further expansion of area under drip/sprinkler technology with the present subsidy criteria. On the other hand, 38% respondents evinced interest in the expansion of area under these technologies even without subsidy. These are the farmers who have realized the advantages of micro-irrigation and needs to be persuaded to act as change agents.

8.4 Suggestions for Effective Implementation

Suggestions based on experiences gained by MIS adopters at farm level are of paramount importance in efficient and satisfactory implementation of MIS. Feedback collected in this regard is provided in Table 8.4.

Frequent power shortage hampered efficient utilization of MIS and associated inputs and accordingly majority of respondents demanded uninterrupted power supply with proper voltage (Table 8.4). Farmers also demanded 50% of the actual cost (market price) of drip set, and its timely release. Other demands included quality material for main set and its spares, timely release of loans from DCCB, effective monitoring, and prompt and satisfactory after sale services. Provision for inbuilt insurance, supply of marketing information, and promotion of in-line discharge system were also suggested by the farmers.

Never the less, similar suggestions were provided by sprinkler adopters. An important suggestion made by the respondents was to supply more nozzles and pipes per set. Respondents requested for effective extension services on regular basis. A quarter of the sprinkler adopters also suggested for making it compulsory and free of cost to marginal and small farmers.

It could be concluded from the above discussions that on the whole respondents were happy with the performance of drip/sprinkler at field level and earned additional income by means of significant savings in critical inputs. Farmers also

Table 8.3
Willingness of Farmers to Extend area under Drip/Sprinkler

S.N.	Particulars	Category		Latur No.	Latur %	Osmanabad No.	Osmanabad %	Total No.	Total %
1	Wish to extend area under drip/sprinkler in future	a) With subsidy	i) Yes	323	89.72	456	81.43	779	84.67
			ii) No	37	10.28	104	18.57	141	15.32
		b) Without subsidy	i) Yes	149	41.39	202	36.07	351	38.15
			ii) No	211	58.61	358	63.93	569	61.85

Source : Field study.

Table 8.4
Suggestions Made by Farmers Using MIS

S.N.	Problem	Drip		
		Latur (n=136)	Osmanabad (n=507)	Total (n=643)
1	Uninterrupted power supply with proper voltage	136 (100.00)	507 (100.00)	643 (100.00)
2	Timely, more amount, and direct subsidy to farmers	128 (94.12)	461 (90.92)	589 (91.60)
3	Quality of drip set and spares should be good	116 (85.29)	472 (93.10)	588 (91.45)
4	Quick, hassle free, and adequate loan facility	120 (88.23)	442 (87.18)	562 (87.40)
5	Subsidy to sand filter and mulching paper	123 (90.44)	433 (85.40)	556 (86.47)
6	Regular technical assistance through training by manufacturers/Govt. officers	101 (74.26)	298 (58.78)	399 (62.05)
7	Prompt and satisfactory after sale services	97 (71.32)	367 (72.38)	464 (72.16)
8	Regular visits and follow ups by dealers and Govt. officers	91 (66.91)	324 (63.90)	415 (64.54)
9	Trouble free system	108 (79.41)	391 (77.12)	499 (77.60)

S.N.	Problem			
10	Reduce price per set	81 (59.56)	252 (49.70)	333 (51.79)
11	Malpractices in implementation of the scheme	53 (38.97)	236 (46.55)	289 (44.94)
12	In-built insurance should be provided	48 (35.29)	202 (39.84)	250 (38.88)
13	Need more marketing information	42 (30.88)	168 (33.14)	210 (32.66)
14	Field verification and monitoring should be strict	87 (63.97)	406 (80.08)	493 (76.67)
15	In-line discharge system should be promoted	38 (27.94)	152 (29.98)	190 (29.55)

Table 8.4 Contd...

S.N.	Problem	Drip		
		Latur (n=224)	Osmanabad (n=53)	Total (n=277)
1	Uninterrupted power supply with proper voltage	224 (100.00)	53 (100.00)	277 (100.00)
2	Timely, more amount, and direct subsidy to farmers	204 (91.07)	47 (88.68)	251 (90.61)
3	Quality of sprinkler set and spares should be good	164 (73.21)	41 (77.36)	205 (74.01)

4	Quick, hassle free, and adequate loan facility	120 (53.57)	27 (50.94)	147 (53.07
5	Sprinkler should be made compulsory and free of cost to small farmers	49 (21.87)	17 (32.07)	66 (23.83)
6	Need better extension services	86 (38.39)	22 (41.51)	108 (39.00)
7	Regular technical assistance through training by manufacturers/Govt. officers	115 (51.34)	30 (56.60)	145 (52.35)
8	Malpractices in implementation of the scheme	94 (41.96)	37 (69.81)	131 (47.30)
9	Provision for more number of nozzles and pipes should be made	186 (83.03)	43 (81.13)	229 (82.67)
10	Prompt and satisfactory after sale services	153 (68.30)	32 (60.38)	185 (66.79)
11	Regular visits, follow ups, and monitoring by dealers and Govt. officers	128 (57.14)	35 (66.04)	163 (58.84)

Figures in brackets indicate percentage to the respective sample size.
Source : Field study.

appreciated efforts of Government in providing subsidy for these capital intensive technologies. They requested to gear up technical and non-technical supports from service providers (manufacturers/dealers) and facilitators (government agency) for effective implementation.

8.5 Summary

An attempt is made in the chapter to highlight the problems faced and future prospects of MIS in the study area. Farmers faced frequent load shedding and hence felt handicapped in efficient utilization of various inputs. High initial costs, delay in subsidy, poor technical assistance from manufactures, etc., were reported by drip adopters. Respondents expected technical assistance from manufacturer/dealers and government agency. Critical loaning procedure and requirement of number of papers consumed valuable time and money. Farmers cultivating cash crops under capital intensive MIS needed trouble-free and quality sets for efficient working of the system on prolonged basis. Interestingly, about 85% sample farmers expressed their willingness for further expansion of area under drip/sprinkler technology with the present subsidy criteria. Farmers appreciated efforts of government in providing subsidy for these capital intensive technologies.

Bibliography

AFC (1998), Evaluation of Drip Irrigation System, Agricultural Finance Corporation (AFC), Ltd., Mumbai.

Bhavanishankar, B.S. (2005), Water Management in India, *Manorama Year Book*, Malayalam Manorama Press, Kottayam: 30.

Chandel, S.S., G.S. Mann, and B. Singh (1997), Marketing of Tomato-Temporal and Spatial Analysis, *Agricultural Marketing*, 40 (2):32-37.

Chopra, K. (1996), The Magnitude of Degraded Land: Issues and Analysis of Technological and Institution Solutions, *Indian Journal of Agricultural Economics*, 51(1&2): 238-248.

CWC (1996), Water and Related Statistics, Ministry of Water Resources, Central Water Commission (CWC), Government of India, New Delhi.

CWC (1998), Water and Related Statistics, Ministry of Water Resources, Central Water Commission (CWC), Government of India, New Delhi.

Dhawan, B.D. (1995), Magnitude of Groundwater Exploitation, *Economic and Political Weekly*, 30(14): 769-775.

Dileep, B.K., R.K. Grover and K.N. Rai (2002), "Contract Farming in Tomato: An Economic Analysis", *Indian Journal of Agricultural Economics*, 57(2):197-210

Dixit, A., R.K. Grover and K.N.Rai (1999), Risk and Uncertainty in Tomato Production: A Case Study of Panipat District in Haryana, *Indian Journal of Agricultural Marketing*, 13(2):59-60.

Ghosh, S. and H.N. Verma (2002), Water in the Twenty-first Century, *Kurukshetra*, 50(3):10-13.

GOI (1992), Report of the Committee on Pricing of Irrigation Water, (Chairman—A. Vaidyanathan), Planning Commission, New Delhi.

GOI (2002), Tenth Five Year Plan: 2002-2007, Vol. II, Planning Commission, New Delhi.

GOM (2003), Economic Survey of Maharashtra, Directorate of Economics and Statistics, Planning Department, Government of Maharashtra, Mumbai.

GOM (2005), Economic Survey of Maharashtra, Directorate of Economics and Statistics, Planning Department, Government of Maharashtra, Mumbai.

INCID (1998), Sprinkler Irrigation in India, Indian National Committee on Irrigation and Drainage, New Delhi.

Kumar, P. and V.C. Mathur (1996), Agriculture in Future: Demand-Supply Perspective for the Ninth-five Year Plan, *Economic and Political Weekly*, 31(29): A131- A139.

MOWR (1999), Report of Working Group on Water Availability for Use, National Commission for Integrated Water Resources Development Plan, Ministry of Water Resources, Government of India, New Delhi.

Narayanamoorthy, A. (1996), Evaluation of Drip Irrigation System in Maharashtra, Mimeograph Series No. 42, Agro-economic Research Centre, GIPE, Pune.

Narayanamoorthy, A. (2001), Impact of Drip Irrigation on Sugarcane Cultivation in Maharashtra, Agro-economic Research Centre, GIPE, Pune.

Narayanamoorthy, A. (2005), Efficiency of Irrigation: A Case

Study of Drip Irrigation, Occasional Paper No. 45, Department of Economic Analysis and Research, NABARD, Mumbai.

Narayanamoorthy, A., and R.S. Deshpande (2003), Irrigation Development and Agricultural Wages: A Analysis Across States, *Economic and Political Weekly*, 38(35): 3716-3722.

Raju, K.V., A. Narayanamoorthy, G. Gopakumar, and H.K. Amarnath (2004), State of the Indian Farmer—A Millennium Study, *Water Resources*, Vol. 3, Ministry of Agriculture, Government of India, New Delhi.

Saleth, R.M. (1996), *Water Institutions in India: Economics, Law and Policy*, Commonwealth Publishers, New Delhi.

Shah, T. (1993), *Groundwater Markets and Irrigation Development, Political Economy and Practical Policy*, Oxford University Press, Delhi.

Sivanappan, R.K. (1994), Micro-irrigation and Macro Future, *Kisan World*, 21(3): 12-15.

Sivanappan, R.K. (1998), Irrigation Water Management for Sugarcane, Vasantdada Sugar Institute: 100-125.

Vaidyanathan, A., A. Krishnakumar, A. Rajgopal and D. Varatharajan (1994), Impact of Irrigation on Productivity of Land, *Journal of Indian School of Political Economy*, 6(4): 601-645.

Index